NUTRITION AND DIET RESEARCH PROGRESS

VITAMIN DEFICIENCY

PREVALENCE, MANAGEMENT AND OUTCOMES

NUTRITION AND DIET RESEARCH PROGRESS

Additional books and e-books in this series can be found on Nova's website under the Series tab.

NUTRITION AND DIET RESEARCH PROGRESS

VITAMIN DEFICIENCY

PREVALENCE, MANAGEMENT AND OUTCOMES

NATALIE STEWART
AND
DAN THOMSON
EDITORS

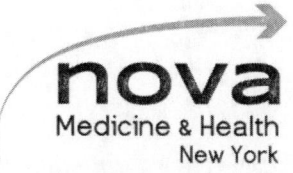

Copyright © 2021 by Nova Science Publishers, Inc.

All rights reserved. No part of this book may be reproduced, stored in a retrieval system or transmitted in any form or by any means: electronic, electrostatic, magnetic, tape, mechanical photocopying, recording or otherwise without the written permission of the Publisher.

We have partnered with Copyright Clearance Center to make it easy for you to obtain permissions to reuse content from this publication. Simply navigate to this publication's page on Nova's website and locate the "Get Permission" button below the title description. This button is linked directly to the title's permission page on copyright.com. Alternatively, you can visit copyright.com and search by title, ISBN, or ISSN.

For further questions about using the service on copyright.com, please contact:
Copyright Clearance Center
Phone: +1-(978) 750-8400   Fax: +1-(978) 750-4470   E-mail: info@copyright.com.

NOTICE TO THE READER

The Publisher has taken reasonable care in the preparation of this book, but makes no expressed or implied warranty of any kind and assumes no responsibility for any errors or omissions. No liability is assumed for incidental or consequential damages in connection with or arising out of information contained in this book. The Publisher shall not be liable for any special, consequential, or exemplary damages resulting, in whole or in part, from the readers' use of, or reliance upon, this material. Any parts of this book based on government reports are so indicated and copyright is claimed for those parts to the extent applicable to compilations of such works.

Independent verification should be sought for any data, advice or recommendations contained in this book. In addition, no responsibility is assumed by the Publisher for any injury and/or damage to persons or property arising from any methods, products, instructions, ideas or otherwise contained in this publication.

This publication is designed to provide accurate and authoritative information with regard to the subject matter covered herein. It is sold with the clear understanding that the Publisher is not engaged in rendering legal or any other professional services. If legal or any other expert assistance is required, the services of a competent person should be sought. FROM A DECLARATION OF PARTICIPANTS JOINTLY ADOPTED BY A COMMITTEE OF THE AMERICAN BAR ASSOCIATION AND A COMMITTEE OF PUBLISHERS.

Additional color graphics may be available in the e-book version of this book.

Library of Congress Cataloging-in-Publication Data

ISBN: 978-1-53618-979-7

Published by Nova Science Publishers, Inc. † New York

CONTENTS

Preface		vii
Chapter 1	The Prevalence and Management of Vitamin D Deficiency among the Pregnant Women and Its Implications: A Global Perspective *Roopa Basutkar Satyanarayan, Pooja Sudarsan and Sivasankaran Ponnusankar*	1
Chapter 2	Study of the Role of Vitamins K and D on the Progression of Human Osteosarcoma Based on *In Vitro* Results *Evangelia Pantazaka, Angelos Kaspiris, Dimitra Melissaridou, Olga D. Savvidou and Panayiotis J. Papagelopoulos*	81
Chapter 3	Implication of Vitamin K in Bone Homeostasis and Osseous Metabolism *Angelos Kaspiris, Efstathios Chronopoulos, Evangelia Pantazaka, Olga D. Savvidou, Elias Vasiliadis and Elias Panagiotopoulos*	103
Index		121

PREFACE

Vitamin Deficiency: Prevalence, Management and Outcomes first assesses the prevalence of vitamin D deficiency and summarizes published randomized controlled studies concerning the supplementation of vitamin D in pregnant women, reporting on the maternal and neonatal outcomes in Asia-Pacific, the United States, Europe, Africa, and the rest of world.

The functions of vitamin K and D are discussed, along with the links between the two vitamins, providing insight on the underlying mechanisms responsible for their role in osteosarcoma and identify future perspectives.

The closing study highlights the vitamin K-dependent biological pathways which are associated with the prevention and treatment of bone metabolism disorders.

Chapter 1 - Globally the prevalence of vitamin D deficiency is around 54% among the pregnant women and is an under diagnosed condition. And as per the Institute of Medicine (IOM), in the pregnant women serum 25(OH)D should be of at least 20 ng/Ml (50 nmol/L). The World Health Organization recommends 200 IU of vitamin D supplementation if pregnant women are vitamin D deficient. Yet, the uncertainties prevail with lack of evidence of recommended dose of vitamin D supplementation during pregnancy. The objective of this part is to assess the prevalence of vitamin D deficiency and summarize the published randomized controlled studies with supplementation of vitamin D among pregnant women and report the maternal and neonatal outcomes in the regions of Asia Pacific, United States of America. Europe, Africa, and Rest of world. The studies both observational and randomized controlled studies published from the year 2005 were identified from PubMed, Scopus, Cochrane CENTRAL and other trial registries. 1,094 citations were identified. Finally, 42 observational studies were identified and 34 randomized and non- randomized clinical trials on its management were identified. Data was extracted using a pre-tested form. The risk of bias of all observational studies was assessed using Newcastle Ottawa scale. Specific scales were used for cross- sectional, cohort, and case- control studies. The Cochrane Collaboration's tool was used for bias assessment of clinical trials. The proportion of vitamin D among pregnant women globally was calculated using the MedCalc statistical software. The effect of Vitamin D supplementation on maternal and neonatal outcomes was measured quantitatively using Review Manager 5.3. The random effect modeling was used for outcomes with high heterogeneity. The quality of evidence for the main outcomes was determined using GradePro. The proportion of vitamin D deficiency during pregnancy was found to be 69.98%, across the globe. The prevalence was found to be 82.4% (95% CI 76.01 to 88.10) for the studies conducted in Asian population when compared with other regions. Maternal 25 (OH) D levels had improved significantly in the vitamin D supplemented group (MD 31.04, 95% CI 21.33 to 40.75). The pooled effect of 25 (OH) D levels were significantly high when administered with ≥2000IU Vitamin D (MD -30.16, 95% CI -37.83 to -22.49) at $p < 0.00001$ ($I^2 = 93\%$). The overall effect of supplementation of vitamin D_3 indicated no difference of developing pre-eclampsia and gestational diabetes in treatment and control group (RR 0.77, 95% CI 0.34 to 1.76) and (RR 0.73, 95% CI 0.51 to 1.06) respectively. The 25 (OH)D levels in cord blood was found to be adequately high in the neonates born to vitamin D_3 supplemented mothers with mean difference of 23.66 (95% CI 13.52 to 33.79, I^2 99%). In conclusion, the prevalence proportion of the vitamin D deficiency is found majorly in Asia. Vitamin D_3 supplementation during pregnancy showed the overall effect in improvement in maternal 25(OH) levels. The 25(OH)D levels in cord blood was found to be high in the neonates born to mothers who were supplemented vitamin D_3 but did not have any significant effect on neonatal anthropometric measures.

Chapter 2 - Osteosarcoma is one of the most prevailing, aggressive primary bone tumors, affecting mainly children and younger populations worldwide. The 60-70% patients' survival rate is not deemed satisfactory, and the high metastasis and relapse frequency, further supports the need for more intense efforts towards the identification of novel therapeutics. Vitamin K, a family of vitamins which exist as both natural and synthetic forms, are essential in bone formation and metabolism and act as cofactor for the post-translational γ-carboxylation of bone matrix proteins. Vitamin K studied in osteosarcoma cells have been reported to be transcriptional regulators of bone-specific genes favoring the expression of bone-related markers, to inhibit cell growth and migration, to induce apoptosis of osteosarcoma cells and affect the transition of cell death mode from apoptosis to necrosis. Vitamin D is another family of fat-soluble vitamins. Vitamin D is known for promoting calcium deposition in bones. Both vitamins K and D have also been demonstrated to exert antitumor effects on a plethora of cancer cell lines, yet their role in osteosarcoma is not fully elucidated. This chapter will introduce these essential vitamins, briefly discuss their functions, present the links between them, provide insight on the underlying mechanisms responsible for their role in osteosarcoma and identify future perspectives.

Chapter 3 - Vitamin K (VK) is a fat-soluble multifunctional vitamin that was originally implicated in blood coagulation. However, current studies elucidate its pivotal role in the maintenance of bone strength, and its positive impact on bone metabolism. VK exerts its anabolic effects on the bone turnover by promoting osteoblast differentiation, by upregulating transcription of specific genes in osteoblasts, and by activating the bone-linked VK dependent proteins that are involved in the mineralization of extracellular bone matrix. Additionally, in vitro studies supported the effects of VK on the differentiation of other mesenchymal stem cells into osteoblasts. Similarly, in vivo experimental studies demonstrated that Steroid and Xenobiotic Receptor (SXR), a putative receptor for vitamin K, is important in the bone homeostasis and metabolism. Several epidemiological surveys revealed that VK status is associated with aging-related musculoskeletal diseases such as osteoporosis, osteoarthritis, and sarcopenia while the combination of vitamin VK and PTH increased the differentiation of osteoblasts appearing synergistic effects on bone formation of bone defects. Furthermore, low VK concentration in the serum was correlated with inflammation and low areal bone mineral density (aBMD) contributing to increased risk of incident fractures. The purpose of this chapter was to highlight the VK-depended biological pathways which are associated to the prevention and treatment of bone metabolism disorders.

In: Vitamin Deficiency ISBN: 978-1-53618-979-7
Editors: N. Stewart and D. Thomson © 2021 Nova Science Publishers, Inc.

Chapter 1

THE PREVALENCE AND MANAGEMENT OF VITAMIN D DEFICIENCY AMONG THE PREGNANT WOMEN AND ITS IMPLICATIONS: A GLOBAL PERSPECTIVE

Roopa Basutkar Satyanarayan[*], *PhD,*
Pooja Sudarsan[†]*, PharmD*
and Sivasankaran Ponnusankar[‡]*, PhD*
Department of Pharmacy Practice, JSS College of Pharmacy,
JSS Academy of Higher Education and Research, Ooty,
The Nilgiris, Tamil Nadu, India

ABSTRACT

Globally the prevalence of vitamin D deficiency is around 54% among the pregnant women and is an under diagnosed condition. And as per the

---

[*] Corresponding Author's E-mail: roopasatyanarayan@gmail.com.
[†] Corresponding Author's E-mail: poojasud96@gmail.com
[‡] Corresponding Author's E-mail: ponnusankarsivas@gmail.com.

Institute of Medicine (IOM), in the pregnant women serum 25(OH)D should be of at least 20 ng/Ml (50 nmol/L). The World Health Organization recommends 200 IU of vitamin D supplementation if pregnant women are vitamin D deficient. Yet, the uncertainties prevail with lack of evidence of recommended dose of vitamin D supplementation during pregnancy. The objective of this part is to assess the prevalence of vitamin D deficiency and summarize the published randomized controlled studies with supplementation of vitamin D among pregnant women and report the maternal and neonatal outcomes in the regions of Asia Pacific, United States of America. Europe, Africa, and Rest of world. The studies both observational and randomized controlled studies published from the year 2005 were identified from PubMed, Scopus, Cochrane CENTRAL and other trial registries. 1,094 citations were identified. Finally, 42 observational studies were identified and 34 randomized and non-randomized clinical trials on its management were identified. Data was extracted using a pre- tested form. The risk of bias of all observational studies was assessed using Newcastle Ottawa scale. Specific scales were used for cross- sectional, cohort, and case- control studies. The Cochrane Collaboration's tool was used for bias assessment of clinical trials. The proportion of vitamin D among pregnant women globally was calculated using the MedCalc statistical software. The effect of Vitamin D supplementation on maternal and neonatal outcomes was measured quantitatively using Review Manager 5.3. The random effect modeling was used for outcomes with high heterogeneity. The quality of evidence for the main outcomes was determined using GradePro. The proportion of vitamin D deficiency during pregnancy was found to be 69.98%, across the globe. The prevalence was found to be 82.4% (95% CI 76.01 to 88.10) for the studies conducted in Asian population when compared with other regions. Maternal 25 (OH) D levels had improved significantly in the vitamin D supplemented group (MD 31.04, 95% CI 21.33 to 40.75). The pooled effect of 25 (OH) D levels were significantly high when administered with ≥2000IU Vitamin D (MD -30.16, 95% CI -37.83 to -22.49) at $p < 0.00001$ ($I^2 = 93\%$). The overall effect of supplementation of vitamin D_3 indicated no difference of developing pre- eclampsia and gestational diabetes in treatment and control group (RR 0.77, 95% CI 0.34 to 1.76) and (RR 0.73, 95% CI 0.51 to 1.06) respectively. The 25 (OH)D levels in cord blood was found to be adequately high in the neonates born to vitamin D_3 supplemented mothers with mean difference of 23.66 (95% CI 13.52 to 33.79, I^2 99%). In conclusion, the prevalence proportion of the vitamin D deficiency is found majorly in Asia. Vitamin D_3 supplementation during pregnancy showed the overall effect in improvement in maternal 25(OH) levels. The 25(OH)D levels in cord blood was found to be high in the neonates born to mothers who were supplemented vitamin D_3 but did not have any significant effect on neonatal anthropometric measures.

Keywords: vitamin D, pregnant women, deficiency, prevalence, management

ABBREVIATIONS

MD	mean difference,
CI	Confidence interval
RR	Risk Ratio
ICTRP	International Clinical Trials Registry Platform.
MeSH	Medical Subject Headings
PS	Pooja Sudarsan
RSB	Roopa Satyanarayan Basutkar
SP	Sivasankaran Ponnusankar
RCT	Randomized Controlled Trial
SD	Standard Deviation.

1. INTRODUCTION

Vitamin D is fat soluble vitamin and the primary source of the vitamin D is from sunlight and food such as fatty fish, eggs, fish liver oil [1]. The vitamin D as supplements are found in forms of vitamin D_2 and D_3. Whereas vitamin D_3 is three time more effective than vitamin D_2 [2]. Both forms of vitamin get hydroxylated to form 25 hydroxyvitamin D in the liver which is in response to the Parathyroid hormone levels [3]. Serum 25(OH)D levels is used to assess the vitamin D levels in body, and this reflects the sum of vitamin D produced cutaneous and obtained in the form of foods and supplements [4]. The Institute of medicine (IOM) defines adequate levels of 25(OH)D levels greater than 50 than 50 nmol/L (or 20 ng/mL) in the pregnant women [5]. The factors that regulate the synthesis and production of vitamin D is skin pigmentation, latitude, dressing codes, season variations and absorption and the metabolism [6]. With respect to skin pigmentation melanin acts a barrier hence reducing the production of vitamin D in the dark-skinned population [7]. People with sedentary lifestyle are less exposed to sunlight and have less levels of 25(OH)D [8]. Population living in the region of high and low latitudes have low levels of 25(OH)D levels. The higher levels of 25 (OH)D is seen during the summer when compared to winter seasons [9]. In the obese population the 25(OH)D gets deposited in body as fat and is stored and its least bioavailable [10].

25(OH)D deficiency is a global health problem and its prevalence is commonly found in infants, pregnant women, and adolescents [11]. Having adequate levels of 25(OH) levels status in the pregnant women is particularly important because the fetus rely on the maternal source for 25 (OH)D levels for their requirement. The requirement of vitamin D during early pregnant is high and continue to increase until delivery. Thus, the maternal vitamin D levels are highly associated with the health outcomes during pregnancy and the infant and neonatal development [12].

Vitamin D deficiency during pregnancy is associated with pre-eclampsia, new onset of gestational hypertension with proteinuria [13], risk for gestational diabetes mellitus [14], linked to caesarean section delivery due to reduced pelvic strength and control and the risk of preterm birth [15]. Due to the maternal 25(OH)D deficiency, the neonates born will have the risk of rickets with osteomalacia, softening of bone, deficiency of phosphorous and calcium [16].

Currently there is no recommendations of supplementing vitamin D during antennal care as per The World Health Organization 2016 statement. The recommendations of vitamin D supplementation to be consumed during the antenatal period differs from each organization. WHO 2004 statement recommends 200 IU/day [17]. Institute of Medicine in the USA recommend 600 IU/day of vitamin D supplementation among the pregnant women[5]. The Royal College of Obstetricians and Gynecologists 2014 statement recommend 400 IU/day and an expert panel in Central Europe recommended 1500 to 2000 IU/day (37.5 to 50.0 mcg/day) [18]. Presently most of the countries do not recommend the use of vitamin D supplement during the routine antenatal care as the evidence present till now is conflicting. Thus the objective of this review is to assess the prevalence of vitamin D deficiency and summarize the published randomized controlled studies with supplementation of vitamin D among pregnant women and report the maternal and neonatal outcomes in the regions of Asia Pacific, United States of America. Europe, Africa, and Rest of world.

2. METHODOLOGY

2.1. Objective

The objective of this chapter is to assess the prevalence of vitamin D deficiency and summarize the published randomized controlled studies on supplementation of vitamin D among pregnant women and report the maternal and neonatal outcomes in the regions of Asia Pacific, United States of America, Europe, Africa, and rest of the world.

2.2. Criteria

2.2.1. Types of Studies

Randomized controlled trials, placebo-controlled trials, and quasi-randomized trials with single or multiple treatment arms were included for analysis. Observational studies on the prevalence of Vitamin D deficiency, maternal and neonatal outcomes of Vitamin D supplementation were also included. Foreign language papers were excluded from review.

2.2.2. Types of Participants

Studies conducted on pregnant women of any demographic characteristics were included for review. Trials that had enrolled participants with pregnancy induced complications or co- morbidities were excluded. Other reasons for exclusion include outcomes reported on post- partum women, infants, and children.

2.2.3. Types of Interventions and Control

We included studies where participants were supplemented with Vitamin D of any dose, frequency, formulation, and duration. Studies comparing higher dose of Vitamin D to lower doses or micro- nutrient supplementation were included.

2.2.4. Types of Outcome Measures

The primary outcome includes the estimation of maternal (maternal 25(OH)D, serum calcium, preeclampsia, gestational diabetes) and neonatal outcomes (anthropometric measures, cord 25 (OH) D) following Vitamin D supplementation. The global prevalence of Vitamin D deficiency among pregnant women was also estimated and presented based on geographical regions. The secondary objectives include the identification of the most effective dose of Vitamin D for pregnant women and the adverse events associated with it.

2.3. Search Methods

2.3.1. Electronic Search

An electronic search was conducted in Cochrane CENTRAL and PubMed using relevant MeSH (Medical Subject Headings) terms from 8th April 2020 to 25th April 2020. Studies published from 2005 were considered for review. Ongoing trials were identified from trial registries such as Clinicaltrials.gov and International Clinical Trials Registry Platform (ICTRP). All queries on missing data were discussed with the respective authors. Handsearching of posters, conference proceedings, in press trials and cross- referencing of included trials favored in identifying studies for inclusion. The keywords used for the search were "Cholecalciferol" or "hydroxycholecalciferols" or "Vitamin D" or "Vitamin D deficiency" or "Pregnancy" or "Perinatal care" or "Vitamin d/therapeutic use" or "Vitamin d/analogs and derivatives" or "dietary supplements" or "pregnancy/drug therapy" or "cholecalciferol/therapy" or "pregnancy complications/ prevention and control."

2.4. Data Collection and Analysis

2.4.1. Selection of Studies
The research articles were search and pooled by two independent reviewers (PS and RSB). The titles and abstracts obtained after literature search were exported to Rayyan to assess its eligibility. Articles were included based on the criteria framed by the researchers. All disagreements were discussed with a third reviewer SP.

2.4.2. Data Extraction and Management
We extracted data using the modified Cochrane data extraction forms for RCT and non- RCT studies. The form was revised to capture details like author details, study design, location, participant demographics, and types of outcome measures, interventions, control, and tools used for outcome measurement. An electronic version of the form was prepared using Excel spreadsheets. The data was entered by two reviewers (PS and RSB) and discrepancies were resolved via discussions with the third reviewer SP.

2.4.3. Risk of Bias Assessment
The risk of bias of all cross- sectional studies addressing the prevalence of Vitamin D deficiency in pregnancy was assessed using Newcastle Ottawa scale. Specific scales were used for cross- sectional, cohort, and case-control studies. Bias was judged by two reviewers (RSB and PS) on three criteria; selection, comparator, and outcome. The Cochrane Collaboration's tool was used for bias assessment of clinical trials. This tool aids in evaluating selection, allocation, blinding, selective reporting, and attrition bias. The judgments were categorized as low, high, or unclear risk. All disagreements were resolved through discussions with SP.

2.4.4. Statistical Analysis
The studies were categorized based on whether they were on prevalence studies or randomized and non- randomized trials on the management of Vitamin D deficiency in pregnancy.

The proportion of vitamin D deficiency among pregnant women globally was calculated using the MedCalc statistical software. The number of events and total number of participants in the vitamin D deficient group was added to the software to obtain a pooled proportion. The level of heterogeneity and statistical significance was also determined. The effect of vitamin D_3 supplementation on maternal and neonatal outcomes was measured quantitatively using Review Manager 5.3. The mean and standard deviation (SD) of continuous outcomes were identified and computed to obtain the forest plot. For outcomes expressed in median and interquartile range, their respective mean ± SD was calculated using the method stated by Hozo et al. [19]. The mean ± SD of multi- arm studies were combined based on the instructions provided in the Cochrane Handbook for Systematic Review. We used random effect modeling for outcomes with high heterogeneity. We had split the primary outcome into several sub- groups to investigate the substantial heterogeneity. The prevalence of Vitamin D deficiency was sub-grouped based on the different geographical regions. Sensitivity analysis was also performed to determine the contribution of each of the studies to the result.

3. RESULTS

3.1. Description of Included Studies

3.1.1. Results of Search

1,094 citations were identified after searching the databases and trial registries. 174 duplicates were removed with 920 records to be screened based on title and abstract. 844 studies were excluded as they did not meet the study criteria. Finally, 42 [20-61] observational studies on the prevalence on Vitamin D deficiency in pregnancy and 34 [62-96] randomized and non-randomized clinical trials on its management were identified.

The prevalence studies were further categorized based on geographical regions as 20 studies from Asia, 13 studies reported from Europe, 2 studies had reported the prevalence in USA and 7 studies from other regions of the world like Canada, Australia and Latin America. The characteristics of the included studies captured the location, latitude, sample size, mean age, vitamin D proportions and risk factors associated with Vitamin D deficiency in pregnancy. Some of the common risk factors were decreased sun exposure, dark pigmentation in skin, lack of prenatal Vitamin D supplementation and seasons (Table 1). Table 2 represents the characteristics of clinical trials conducted on Vitamin D supplementation in pregnancy. The dose and duration of Vitamin D supplements, maternal and neonatal outcomes associated with it as depicted in the Table.

3.1.2. Quality Assessment of Included Studies

3.1.2.1. Observational Studies

Out of the 42 observational studies, the risk of bias was identified in cross- sectional studies. Sample size was not calculated in 12 studies (Agarwal 2016, Fareed 2019, Hong-Bi 2018, Kaur 2019, Nageshu 2016, Ocal 2019, Prasad 2018, Pratumvinit 2015, Sachan 2005, Sharma 2019, Shrestha 2019 and Yadav 2018 [20, 25, 27-30, 32-36, 38]. No information on the use of validated tool for measuring outcomes and response rate in comparators were provided by Fareed 2019. Hence, the overall risk assessment score was high for the cross- sectional study by Fareed et al. [25]. A comparison group was not used in the studies by Kaur 2019, Nageshu 2016, Ocal 2019 and Prasad 2018 [28-30, 32]. Five cross- sectional studies (Agarwal 2016, Fareed 2019, Kaur 2019, and Yadav 2018) [20, 25, 28] had used only descriptive statistical tests to present their results. The bias assessment of cross- sectional studies is represented by a stacked graph (Figure 2).

Table 1. Characteristics of observational studies on the prevalence of Vitamin D deficiency in pregnancy

Study ID (Author, year)	Country + Latitude	Study design	Sample size	Mean age (years)	Vitamin D cut off points	Assay method	Prevalence rate	Factors
ASIA								
Agarwal et al., 2016	Surat, India	Cross-Sectional	253	NA	Deficient: <20 ng/ml, Insufficient: 21-29 ng/ml, Sufficient: ≥30 ng/ml	NA	Deficient: 83.4% Insufficient: 11.1% Sufficient: 5.53%	Low socio-economic status (94%), obesity (100%), anemia (86%), pregnancy-induced hypertension (93%) and gestational diabetes mellitus (83%).
Aji et al., 2019	Indonesia	Cross-Sectional	239	29.77 ± 5.68	Deficient: <12 ng/mL) Sufficient: ≥20 ng/mL), Insufficient: 12–19 ng/mL	ELISA	Deficient: 82.8% Sufficient: 17.2%	No working status (OR: 0.02), nulliparity (OR: 7.6), outdoor activity less than 1 hour (OR: 9.6) and no prenatal consumption of supplements (OR: 4.49)
Aly et al., 2013	Saudi Arabia	Case control	118	33 ± 6.2	Deficient: <30 nmol/L, Insufficient: 30-50 nmol/L, Sufficient: >50 nmol/L	EIA	Deficient: 14.2% Insufficient: 50% Sufficient: 35.8%	Low sun exposure (52%), multiparity (49%), low socio-economic status (57%) and living in rural area (54%).
Charatcharoenwitthaya et al., 2013	Thailand	Cross-sectional study	120	29.3 ± 5.7	Inadequacy: <75 nM, Insufficiency: 50 and 75 nM, Deficient: <50 nM	LC-MS/MS	Deficiency 1st trimester: 83.3% 2nd trimester: 30.9% 3rd trimester: 27.4%	Not taking prenatal supplements (OR: 9.70), first trimester (OR: 10.58) and not drinking vitamin fortified milk (OR: 11.42).

Study ID (Author, year)	Country + Latitude	Study design	Sample size	Mean age (years)	Vitamin D cut off points	Assay method	Prevalence rate	Factors
ASIA								
Choi et al., 2015	South Korea (latitude 36°N)	Cross-sectional study	220	Median age was 32	Sufficient: ≥30 ng/mL (≥75 nmol/L) Suboptimal: 20–29.9 ng/mL(50–74.9 nmol/L)	LC-MS/MS	Deficient: 77.3% Severe deficiency: 28.6%	First trimester (OR: 4.3), winter: 100%.
Fareed et al., 2019	Srinagar, India	Observational study	50	21-25	NA	LC-MS/MS	Deficient: 68%	No consumption of multivitamins (38%), less than half an hour sun exposure (26%) and smoking (18%).
Ganmaa et al., 2014	Mongolia, China	Cross-sectional	420	34.9 ± 4.8	Deficient: ≤20 ng/ml	LC-MS/MS	Deficient: 98.8% Inadequate: <1% Sufficient: 0.2%	Educational status and use of vitamin D supplements.
Hong-Bi et al., 2018	Guizhou, China	Cross-sectional study	220	29.3 ± 4.5	Deficient: <30 nmol/L (<12 ng/mL), Inadequate: 30 to 50 nmol/L (12 to 20 ng/mL), Sufficient: >50 nmol/L (>20 ng/mL)	ELISA	Deficient: 72.3% Inadequate: 20.5% Sufficient: 7.3%	Prevalence of vitamin D deficiency was high in participants with adverse perinatal outcomes.

Table 1. (Continued)

Study ID (Author, year)	Country + Latitude	Study design	Sample size	Mean age (years)	Vitamin D cut off points	Assay method	Prevalence rate	Factors
ASIA								
Kaur et al, 2019	Jammu, India	Cross-sectional study	120	NA	Deficient: <20 ng/ml(<50 nmol/L), Insufficient: 20-30 ng/ml (50 to 75 nmol/L), Sufficient: >30 ng/ml (>75 nmol/L)	CLIA	Deficient: 43.3% Insufficient: 34.1% Sufficient: 22.5%	Increase in maternal age
Nageshu et al, 2016	Andhra Pradesh, India	Cross-Sectional	80	18-35	NA	EIA	Deficient: 13.8% Insufficient: 53.8%	1 to 2 hours of sun exposure (65.1%)
Ocal et al, 2019	Turkey	Cross-Sectional	600	Study group: 18.43 ± 1.30 Control group: 28.67 ± 5.38	NA	ELISA	Deficient: 86%	Winter (98%) and level of education
Özdemir et al, 2018	Turkey	Cross-Sectional	120	20 to ≥30	Deficient: <12 ng/mL (<30 nmol/L), Insufficient: 12-20 ng/mL (30-50 nmol/L), Sufficient: >20 ng/mL (>50 nmol/L)	Enzyme linked fluorescent assay	Deficient: 49.5% Insufficient: 36.1% Sufficient: 14.4%	Daily vitamin D intake and clothing style.

Study ID (Author, year)	Country + Latitude	Study design	Sample size	Mean age (years)	Vitamin D cut off points	Assay method	Prevalence rate	Factors
ASIA								
Prasad et al., 2018	Bihar, India	Cross-sectional	100	30	Deficient: < 20ng/ml, Insufficient: 20-30ng/ml, Sufficient: 30-100ng/ml	NA	Deficient: 88%	Housewife (86%) and multiparity (68%).
Pratumvinit et al, 2015	Bangkok, Thailand Latitude 13.45°N.	Cross-sectional study	147	28.9 ± 6.4	Sufficient: ≥75, Hypovitaminosis D <75, Insufficient: 50-74.9, Deficient: <50	Electro-chemiluminescence immunoassay	Hypovitaminosis D: 75.5% Insufficient: 41.5% Deficient: 34%	Lower pre-pregnancy BMI (OR: 0.88) and winter (OR: 2.62)
Sachan et al., 2005	Lucknow, India, 26.8°N	Cross-sectional study	207	24.0 ± 4.1	NA	RIA	Hypovitaminosis D: 84% <10ng/mL: 42.5% <15ng/mL: 66.7%	Maternal vitamin D levels had positive correlation with cord vitamin D levels and negative correlation with parathyroid hormone levels.
Sharma et al., 2019	Meghalaya, India	Cross-sectional study	177	26.71 ± 9.96	Deficient: <20 ng/mL, Insufficient: <32 ng/mL	NA	Deficient: 84.18% Insufficient: 12.44%	Parity and pregnancy induced hypertension
Shrestha et al., 2019	Bhaktapur, Nepal	Cross-sectional study	106	26.7 ± 4.7	Deficient: < 20 ng/ml, Insufficient: 20–30 ng/ml	Fluorescence immunoassay	Deficient: 81%	NA

Table 1. (Continued)

Study ID (Author, year)	Country + Latitude	Study design	Sample size	Mean age (years)	Vitamin D cut off points	Assay method	Prevalence rate	Factors
ASIA								
Woon et al., 2019	Malaysia Selangor: 3.074° N and Kuala Lumpur: 3.139° N	Cohort	535	29.9 ± 4.1	Deficient: < 30 nmol/L, Insufficient: 30–50 nmol/L, Sufficient: 50 nmol/L	Vitamin D Total assay	Deficient: 42.6% Insufficient: 49.4% Sufficient: 8%	Intake of vitamin D supplements (OR: 0.96) and non- Malaysians (OR: 0.14)
Yadav et al., 2018	Rajasthan, India	Observational study	120	Deficient group 28.31 ± 3.86 Sufficient group 26.37 ± 2.83	Not defined	CLIA and RIA	Deficient: 84.1%	Use of sun screen lotion and vegetarian diet
Yun et al., 2015	China	Cross-sectional	1985	The median age of the participants was 26·10	10 and 15 µg/d for 25(OH)D concentrations of 16 and 20 ng/ml, respectively	EIA	Deficient: 74.9%	Lack of consumption of vitamin D supplements, Hui ethnicity and low ambient UVB levels
EUROPE								
Brembeck et al., 2013	Sweden (Latitudes 57–58°N)	Cross-sectional	95	32·2 years	Not mentioned	CLIA	<30 nmol/L: 17% 30- 49.9 nmol/L: 48% ≥50 nmol/L: 35%	Season, travel to Southern latitudes, use of vitamin D supplements, use of sun screen and skin color

Study ID (Author, year)	Country + Latitude	Study design	Sample size	Mean age (years)	Vitamin D cut off points	Assay method	Prevalence rate	Factors
EUROPE								
Cabaset et al., 2019	Switzerland	Cross-sectional	204	30.03 ± 4.85	Women with serum 25(OH)D concentrations above 20 ng/mL were considered as non-deficient (which includes both insufficient (20 to 30 ng/mL) and sufficient (above 30 ng/mL) as defined by the Endocrine Society	Electro-chemo-luminescence immunoassay	Deficient: 63.2%	Non- smokers, lack of vitamin D intake and country of origin (other than Switzerland and Germany)
Dovnik et al., 2014	Slovenia	Cross-sectional	100	NA	Severe deficiency: <25 nmol/L Deficient: 25–50 nmol/L Insufficiency: 50–80 nmol/L Optimal: >80 nmol/L	Electro-chemiluminescence immunoassay	Severe deficiency (December group): 40% Severe deficiency (September group): 10%	Lack of vitamin D intake
Emmerson et al., 2016	United Kingdom	Cross-sectional	630	Median (IQR) 31.4 (27.9–34.8)	Deficiency: <25 nmol/L Insufficiency: <50 nmol/L	LC-MS/MS	Deficient: 7% Insufficient: 27% Sufficient: 73%	White skinned women with Fitzpatrick skin-type I

Table 1. (Continued)

Study ID (Author, year)	Country + Latitude	Study design	Sample size	Mean age (years)	Vitamin D cut off points	Assay method	Prevalence rate	Factors
EUROPE								
Haggarty et al., 2013	Scotland (latitude 57°N)	Prospective Cohort	1205	30·7 ± 5·3	NA	liquid chromatography–tandem MS (LC-MS/MS) after	<25nmol/L: 21.5%	Season, vitamin D diet and supplementation
Holmes et al., 2009	Belfast, United Kingdom 54–55°N.	longitudinal study	120	28·8 ± 5·6	Severe deficiency: 12·5 nmol/l Deficiency: 25 nmol/l Insufficiency: 50 nmol/l and 80 nmol/l	ELISA	Deficient (12 weeks of gestation): 35% Deficient (20 weeks of gestation): 44% Deficient (35 weeks of gestation): 16%	Inadequate dose of vitamin D supplementation
Jóźwiak et al., 2014	Poland	Cross-sectional	88	30.68 ± 4.82	Definition of vitamin D deficiency and insufficiency was based on the Endocrine Society's Practice Guidelines on Vitamin D	Electro-chemiluminescence immunoassay	Deficient: 31.8% Insufficient: 26.1% Sufficient: 42%	Lack of consumption of vitamin D supplements
Krieger et al., 2018	Zurich, Bellinzona, Samedan	Cross-sectional	305	32·9 ± 5.2	Deficiency: <50 nmol/l Sufficiency: ≥50 nmol/L	Electro-chemiluminescence immunoassay	Deficient: 53.4%	Season, intake of vitamin D supplements and country of origin

Study ID (Author, year)	Country + Latitude	Study design	Sample size	Mean age (years)	Vitamin D cut off points	Assay method	Prevalence rate	Factors
EUROPE								
Lundqvist et al., 2016	Sweden, (latitude 63.8° N)	Cohort	226	31 ± 4.4	Vitamin D insufficiency has been defined as serum vitamin D levels of <50 nmol/L	Liquid chromatography-tandem mass spectrometry (LC-MS/MS)	Deficient (12 weeks of gestation): 35% Deficient (21 weeks of gestation): 34.6% Deficient (35 weeks of gestation): 28.7%	Multivitamin use and seasons
McAree et al., 2013	United Kingdom	Retrospective study	4799	NA	Deficiency: equal to or under 25 nmol/L, Insufficiency: 25–74 nmol/L Adequacy: ≥ 75 nmol/L	LC-MS	Deficient: 36% Insufficient: 45% Adequate: 18%	Skin tone (only 8% of dark skinned mothers had adequate levels)
Nicolaidou et al., 2006	Greece	Observational study	139	Median age (IQR) was 28 (24, 32) years	NA	CLIA (two site)	<10ng/mL: 19.5%	Dark phenotype and seasons (winter and spring)
Rodriguez et al., 2016	Spain	Cohort	2150	NA	Deficient: <20 ng/mL Insufficiency: 20–30 ng/mL Optimal: >30 ng/mL,	HPLC	Insufficient: 31% Deficient: 18%	Low socio-economic status (RR: 1.94) and smoking (RR: 1.76)

Table 1. (Continued)

Study ID (Author, year)	Country + Latitude	Study design	Sample size	Mean age (years)	Vitamin D cut off points	Assay method	Prevalence rate	Factors
EUROPE								
Vandevijvere et al., 2012	Brussels, Flanders Wallonia Belgium	Cross-sectional	1311	28.5 ± 5.1	Severely deficient: <10ng/mL Deficient: <20ng/mL Insufficient: <30ng/mL	RIA	Severely deficient: 12.1% Deficient: 44.6% Insufficient: 74.1%	Sun exposure, smoking status, low education status
OTHER REGIONS								
Davies-Tuck et al., 2015	Australia	Cross-sectional	1550	30 ± 5.4	Deficient: <50nmol/L Insufficient: 50-75nmol/L Replete: ≥75nmol/L	CLIA	Deficient: 55% Insufficient: 37% Replete: 8%	Winter or spring (50%), BMI ≥36kg/m² (OR: 2.6), Country of birth (South-East, Southern or Eastern Asia, Africa more likely to be deficient)
Figueiredo et al., 2018	Rio de Janeiro, Brazil	Prospective Cohort	299	26.6 ± 5.5	Deficient: <50 nmol/L Insufficient: 50-75 nmol/L Sufficient: ≥75 nmol/L	Liquid chromatography–tandem mass spectrometry (LC–MS/MS)	Deficient (5th to 13th weeks of gestation): 16.1% Deficient (20th to 26th weeks of gestation): 11.2% Deficient (30th to 36th weeks of gestation): 10.2%	Seasonal variation

Study ID (Author, year)	Country + Latitude	Study design	Sample size	Mean age (years)	Vitamin D cut off points	Assay method	Prevalence rate	Factors
Jones et al., 2016	Western Australia	Cross-sectional	209	32.8 ± 4.4	Deficient: <50 nmol/l), Insufficient: 50 to <75 nmol/l Sufficient: ≥75 nmol/l	CLIA	Deficient: 13.9%	Ambient UV radiation (OR: 2.82),
OTHER REGIONS								
Kramer et al., 2016	Toronto, Canada	Cohort study	467	Deficient: 34.2 ± 4.3 Insufficient:34.5 ± 4.2 Sufficient: 34.3 ± 4.3	Deficient: < 50 nmol/l) Insufficient: 50 to 75 nmol/l) Sufficient: ≥75 nmol/l)	Electro-chemiluminescence immunoassay	Deficient: 31.5% Insufficient: 35.1%	Seasons and intake of vitamin D supplements
Perreault et al., 2019	Ontario, Canada	Cohort	332	32.5 ± 4.7	NA	Ultra-performance liquid chromatography tandem mass spectrometry (UPLC-MS/MS)	NA	European descent and summer season were associated with vitamin D sufficiency
Shand et al., 2010	Vancouver, British Columbia, Canada (49°N)	Prospective cohort study.	221	18 to ≥ 35 years	Deficient: <50nmol/L Insufficient: <75nmol/L	RIA	Deficient: 53% Insufficient: 78%	NA

Table 1. (Continued)

Study ID (Author, year)	Country + Latitude	Study design	Sample size	Mean age (years)	Vitamin D cut off points	Assay method	Prevalence rate	Factors
Wei et al., 2012	Canada	Prospective cohort study.	697	Pre-eclamptic: 30.9 ± 5.3 Non-preeclamptic: 30.3 ± 4.8	Deficient: <50 nmol/l	CLIA	Deficient: 39%	Vitamin D deficiency was significantly associated with pre-eclampsia (OR: 3.24)
OTHER REGIONS								
Hamilton et al., 2010	South Carolina at, USA Latitude 32°N	Cross-sectional	1559	25.0 ± 5.4	Deficiency: <20 ng/mL (<50 nmol/L) and Insufficiency: 20 and 32 ng/mL (50–80 nmol/L)	RIA	<12ng/mL: 15.8% 12- 19ng/mL: 32.2% 20- 31ng/mL: 37.1% ≥32ng/mL: 14.9%	Dark pigmentation increases the risk of Vitamin D deficiency
Luque-Fernandez et al., 2013	USA	Cohort	2583	15 to ≥35	NA	Liquid chromatography-tandem mass spectrometry	NA	Non- Hispanic black women and seasonal variation

NA: Not Available, ELISA: Enzyme Linked Immunosorbent Assay, OR: Odds Ratio, EIA: Immunodiagnostic enzyme immuno-assay, LS-MS/MS: Liquid chromatography–tandem mass spectrometry, CLIA: Chemiluminescent Immunoassay, RIA: Radioimmunoassay, BMI: Body Mass Index, HPLC: High Performance Liquid Chromatography, RR: Risk Ratio.

Table 2. Characteristics of the included clinical trials on the management of Vitamin D deficiency in pregnancy

Study ID	Country	Study Design	Trimester (weeks of gestation)	Mean age (years)	No. of participants	Intervention (With dose)	Control (With dose)	Duration	Maternal Outcomes	Neonatal Outcomes	Vitamin D cut offs and unit of measurement
ASIA											
Ali et al., 2019	Riyadh, Saudi Arabia	Open labeled randomized controlled study	6-12	20-40	179	4000 IU vitamin D3 (40 drops daily)	Multivitamin-Multimineral Supplement containing 400 IU vitamin D3/tablet once daily	13 weeks-12 weeks post-partum	Pre-eclampsia, Total 25(OH)D, IUGR	Birth weight	Deficiency: <25 nmol/L, Insufficiency: 25-75 nmol/L, Sufficiency: 75-200 nmol/L and Toxicity:>250 nmol/L
Asemi et al., 2013	Kashan, Iran	Randomized, double-blind, placebo-controlled clinical trial	25	18-40	48	400 IU/d cholecalciferol	Placebo	9 week	Serum25(OH)D, hs-CRP, SBP and DBP, FPG, Lipid profiles, Calcium	NA	NA
Dawodu et al., 2013	United Arab Emirates	Randomized controlled double-blind study	12-16	25-27	192	400IU and 2000IU vitamin D3	400IU vitamin D3	40 day supply of study drugs and 90 day supply of prenatal vitamin (400IU)	Serum25(OH)D Serum calcium iPTH	Cord 25(OH)D	Sufficiency: 32 ng/ml

Table 2. (Continued)

Study ID	Country	Study Design	Trimester (weeks of gestation)	Mean age (years)	No. of participants	Intervention (With dose)	Control (With dose)	Duration	Maternal Outcomes	Neonatal Outcomes	Vitamin D cut offs and unit of measurement
ASIA											
Enkhmaa et al., 2019	Mongolia	Randomized, controlled, double-blind trial	12–16	≥18	360	600, 2000, or 4000 IU vitamin D₃	NA	12 weeks of gestation until delivery	Serum25(OH)D, Serum calcium	Cord blood 25(OH)D concentrations	NA
Hashemipour et al., 2014	Qazvin (Iran)	Open-label randomized clinical trial	24–26	26–27	130	200 mg calcium plus a multivitamin (containing vitamin D3 400 U) each day + vitamin D3 (50,000 IU) each week	200 mg calcium plus a multivitamin (containing vitamin D3 400 U) each day	8 weeks	Serum25(OH)D, Maternal weight gain	Cord blood 25(OH)D concentrations, anthropometric measures	Deficiency: <20 ng/ml Insufficiency: 20–30 ng/ml
Hossain et al., 2014	Karachi, Pakistan	Single center, open label, randomized controlled trial	20	25	200	Ferrous sulfate 200 mg, twice daily and 600mg of calcium lactate daily + 4000 IU of vitamin D3 drops	Ferrous sulfate 200 mg, twice daily and 600mg of calcium lactate daily	20 weeks to delivery	Serum25(OH)D, Gestational hypertension, Glucose challenge test, Pre-eclampsia, GDM, Pre-term birth	Serum25(OH)D, Anthropometric parameters, SGA	Deficiency: <30ng/mL Severe deficiency: ≤10ng/mL

Study ID	Country	Study Design	Trimester (weeks of gestation)	Mean age (years)	No. of participants	Intervention (With dose)	Control (With dose)	Duration	Maternal Outcomes	Neonatal Outcomes	Vitamin D cut offs and unit of measurement
ASIA											
Kalra et al., 2012	Lucknow, India	Prospective, partially Randomized Controlled trial	12–24	25–26	299	Calcium carbonate 1g + One oral dose of 1500mg vitamin D3 'or' Two doses of 3000mg vitamin D3	Calcium carbonate 1g without vitamin D	To delivery	Serum25(OH)D	Serum25(OH)D, ALP, Anthropometric parameters, Serum calcium	NA
Karamali et al., 2015	Arak, Iran	Randomized double-blind placebo-controlled clinical trial	20–32	18–40	60	50 000 IU vitamin D (Cholecalciferol)	Placebo	12 weeks	Serum25(OH)D, HOMA-IR, FPG Lipid profile, Pre-eclampsia rate, Inflammatory biomarkers	Anthropometric parameters	NA
Mojibian et al., 2015	Yazd, Iran	Randomized clinical trial	12–16	27	500	50,000 IU vitamin D (Cholecalciferol)	400 IU vitamin D (Cholecalciferol)	12 weeks until delivery	Serum25(OH)D, GDM, FPG, Pre-eclampsia	Cord blood 25(OH)D, Anthropometric parameters, Neonatal complication (Macrosomia, hypoglycemia etc.)	NA

Table 2. (Continued)

Study ID	Country	Study Design	Trimester (weeks of gestation)	Mean age (years)	No. of participants	Intervention (With dose)	Control (With dose)	Duration	Maternal Outcomes	Neonatal Outcomes	Vitamin D cut offs and unit of measurement
ASIA											
Motamed et al., 2019	Tehran, Iran	Open-label randomized clinical trial	<12	18–40	84	1,000-IU/d vitamin D or 2,000 IU/d vitamin D	NA	12 weeks until delivery	Serum25(OH)D, hs-CRP, cell-culture supernatant concentrations of IL-1β, IL-6, and TNF-α, Preeclampsia, GDM, Urinary Calcium/Creatinine ratio	Cord blood 25(OH)D, Anthropometric parameters, hs-CRP, IL-1β, IL-6, TNF-α	Deficiency: <50 nmol/L Insufficiency: 50–75 nmol/L Sufficiency: >75 nmol/L
Rostami et al., 2018	Iran	Randomized placebo clinical trial	<14	18 to 40	800	Group A1/B1: treated with 50,000 IU of oral D3 weekly for a total duration of 12 weeks. Group A2/B2: treated with 50,000 IU of oral D3 weekly for a total duration of 12 weeks plus a monthly maintenance dose of 50,000 IU of D3 until delivery. Group A3/B3: treated with intramuscular administration of 300,000 IU of D3 each 6 weeks for two doses			Serum 25(OH)D, Pre-eclampsia, GDM, Preterm delivery	NA	Moderate: 10 to 20 ng/mL Severe: 10 ng/mL

Study ID	Country	Study Design	Trimester (weeks of gestation)	Mean age (years)	No. of participants	Intervention (With dose)	Control (With dose)	Duration	Maternal Outcomes	Neonatal Outcomes	Vitamin D cut offs and unit of measurement
							Group A4/B4: treated with intramuscular administration of 300,000 IU of D3 each 6 weeks for 2 doses plus monthly maintenance dose of 50,000 IU of D3 until delivery.				

ASIA

Study ID	Country	Study Design	Trimester (weeks of gestation)	Mean age (years)	No. of participants	Intervention (With dose)	Control (With dose)	Duration	Maternal Outcomes	Neonatal Outcomes	Vitamin D cut offs and unit of measurement
Roth et al., 2013	Bangladesh	Randomized placebo-controlled trial	26 to 29	18 to <35	160	35,000 IU	Placebo	12 weeks	25(OH)D, Calcium, Albumin-adjusted calcium, PTH, Urinary calcium-creatinine ratio	25(OH)D, Calcium, Albumin-adjusted calcium, PTH, Urinary calcium-creatinine ratio	NA
Roth et al., 2018	Bangladesh	Randomized, double-blind, placebo-controlled	17 to 24	≥18	1300	3 Groups 4200 IU 16800 IU 28000 IU	Placebo	12 Weeks	25(OH)D, Calcium, PTH, Urinary calcium-creatinine ratio	Serum 25(OH)D	Deficiency below 30 nmol Per liter (<12 ng per milliliter).

Table 2. (Continued)

Study ID	Country	Study Design	Trimester (weeks of gestation)	Mean age (years)	No. of participants	Intervention (With dose)	Control (With dose)	Duration	Maternal Outcomes	Neonatal Outcomes	Vitamin D cut offs and unit of measurement
Sablok et al., 2015	India	Randomize controlled trail	20 and 24	NA	180	Based on Serum 25(OH)D dose is Deficient: 480000IU Insufficient: 240000 IU Sufficient: 60000 IU	NA	20 weeks	Serum 25(OH)D	Serum 25(OH)D	Sufficient: >50nmol/L, Insufficient: 25-50nmol/L and Deficient: <25nmol/L.
ASIA											
Sahoo et al., 2017	India	A double-blind, randomized, placebo-controlled, multi-arm parallel study	14 to 20	>18	300 (1:1:1)	Group 1: 60,000IU every 4 weeks Group 2: 60,000IU every 8 weeks	Placebo	Till delivery	Serum 25(OH)D	Cord blood 25(OH)D	NA
Sahu et al., 2009	India	Pilot interventional study	Second trimester	NA	84	Group B: 60000 IU Group C: 120,000 IU	NA	Group B: 5th month Group C: 5th and 7th month	Serum 25(OH)D, Calcium	NA	NA

Study ID	Country	Study Design	Trimester (weeks of gestation)	Mean age (years)	No. of participants	Intervention (With dose)	Control (With dose)	Duration	Maternal Outcomes	Neonatal Outcomes	Vitamin D cut offs and unit of measurement
Shakiba et al., 2013	Iran	Randomized study	Second trimester	NA	51	Group A: 50,000IU/month, Group B:1,00,000 IU/month Group C: 2,00,000+ 50,000IU/month	NA	Till delivery	Serum 25(OH)D	Cord blood 25(OH)D	Cord blood of neonates: Sufficient: > 30 ng/mL Insufficient: 20–30 ng/mL Deficient: < 20 ng/mL
ASIA											
Vafaei et al., 2019	Iran	Randomized study	Two weeks after menstrual retardation	20–35 years	140	1000 IU	Placebo	Till 34 weeks of gestation	Serum 25OHD	Sonographic data	Deficient: < 20 ng/mL, Insufficient: 20–30 ng/mL Sufficient: > 30 ng/mL
Vaziri et al., 2016	Iran	Randomized placebo controlled trial	26-28	≥18	134	2000 IU	Placebo	Till delivery	Serum 25(OH)D	Anthropometric measurements	NA
Yesiltepe Mutlu et al., 2014	Turkey	Randomized controlled trial	13 to 32	>16	120	600 IU 1000 IU 2000 IU	No control group	NA	Serum 25(OH)D, Serum Calcium	Serum 25(OH)D, Serum Calcium, Birth weight	Serum 25(OH)D <20 ng/ml

Table 2. (Continued)

Study ID	Country	Study Design	Trimester (weeks of gestation)	Mean age (years)	No. of participants	Intervention (With dose)	Control (With dose)	Duration	Maternal Outcomes	Neonatal Outcomes	Vitamin D cut offs and unit of measurement
EUROPE											
Cooper et al., 2016	UK (Southampton, Oxford, and Sheffield)	Multicenter, double-blind, randomized, placebo-controlled trial	14	>18	1134	Cholecalciferol 1000IU/day	Placebo	14 weeks till delivery	Serum 25(OH)D	Whole-body BMC, neonatal whole-body bone area, BMD, size-corrected BMC, body composition	NA
EUROPE											
Corcoy et al., 2020	Seven European countries (UK, Ireland, Austria, Poland, Italy (Padua, Pisa), Spain, and Belgium)	Randomized factorial design	<19 weeks+6 days of gestation	≥18	154	Vitamin D 1600IU/day	Placebo	<19 weeks until delivery	Total 25(OH)D, Serum Calcium, Urinary calcium, Pre-eclampsia, FPG, Insulin sensitivity (HOMA- IR), GWG, PIH, Weight gain	Total 25(OH)D, Preterm birth, Birth weight, APGAR score	Threshold ≥50 nmol/l

Study ID	Country	Study Design	Trimester (weeks of gestation)	Mean age (years)	No. of participants	Intervention (With dose)	Control (With dose)	Duration	Maternal Outcomes	Neonatal Outcomes	Vitamin D cut offs and unit of measurement
Moon et al., 2016	UK	Double-blind, multicenter, randomized, placebo-controlled trial (MAVIDOS)	<17	>18	1134	1000 IU/d of cholecalciferol + Dietary supplements of 400IU/d vitamin D	Placebo + Dietary supplements of 400IU/d vitamin D	14 weeks until delivery	Serum25(OH), Weight gain	NA	NA
EUROPE											
O'Callaghan et al., 2018	Cork, Ireland (51.9° N)	3-arm, dose-response, parallel double-blind, randomized placebo-controlled trial	3 time points 1) Baseline: 8–18 week 2) Mid-gestation: 20–26 week 3) Late gestation: 34–38 week	21 to 41	144	10µg (400 IU) or 20µg (800 IU) vitamin D3/d	Placebo	18 weeks	Total 25(OH)D, Serum calcium, iPTH	Total 25(OH)D, Serum calcium, iPTH	Umbilical cord 25(OH)D threshold: ≥25–30 nmol/L

Table 2. (Continued)

Study ID	Country	Study Design	Trimester (weeks of gestation)	Mean age (years)	No. of participants	Intervention (With dose)	Control (With dose)	Duration	Maternal Outcomes	Neonatal Outcomes	Vitamin D cut offs and unit of measurement
Stoutjesdijk et al., 2018	Netherlands	Randomized trial	20	NA	43	0, 25, 50 and 75 µg vitamin D3	NA	4 weeks post-partum	Serum 25(OH)D, Milk ARA	NA	Deficiency: <25nmol/L, Insufficiency: 25-49 nmol/L, Sufficiency: 80-249nmol/L Toxicity: >250 nmol/L
Yu et al., 2009	London, UK	Randomized study	27	NA	180	Group 1: A daily dose of vitamin D (ergocalciferol) at 800 IU Group 2: A stat dose of 2,00,000 IU of (calciferol)	NA	Till delivery	Serum 25(OH)D, PTH, Serum Calcium	Cord 25(OH)D	Sufficiency: ≥50 nmol/l, Insufficiency: 25–50 nmol/l Deficiency: <25 nmol/l.

Study ID	Country	Study Design	Trimester (weeks of gestation)	Mean age (years)	No. of participants	Intervention (With dose)	Control (With dose)	Duration	Maternal Outcomes	Neonatal Outcomes	Vitamin D cut offs and unit of measurement
USA AND CANADA											
Hollis et al., 2011	South Carolina, USA	Single-center, randomized, controlled, double blind study	12 to 16	≥16	494	Standard prenatal multivitamin vitamin containing 400 IU of vitamin D + All patients received a total of two pills daily: 2000 IU, or 4000 IU of vitamin D3	Standard prenatal multivitamin vitamin containing 400 IU of vitamin D	12 weeks until delivery	Serum25(OH)D, Serum calcium, iPTH, Urinary Calcium/Creatinine ratio	Serum25(OH)D, Birth-weight	Deficiency: <50nmol/L Insufficiency:50nmol/L- 80nmol/L Sufficiency: >80nmol/L
March et al., 2015	British Columbia, Canada	Double-blind randomized controlled trial	13- 24	18-45	226	10, 25, or 50 mg/d of vitamin D	NA	8 weeks post-partum	Serum25(OH)D, Serum calcium, Urinary Calcium/Creatinine ratio	Cord blood 25(OH)D	Deficient: 30 nmol/L Average requirement: 40 nmol/L Meet/ exceed the needs: 50 nmol/L Canadian Pediatric Society recommendation: 75 nmol/L

Table 2. (Continued)

Study ID	Country	Study Design	Trimester (weeks of gestation)	Mean age (years)	No. of participant	Intervention (With dose)	Control (With dose)	Duration	Maternal Outcomes	Neonatal Outcomes	Vitamin D cut offs and unit of measurement
USA AND CANADA
Thiele et al., 2017	Portland, USA	Double-blind, randomized controlled trial	24 to 28	≥18	16	Prenatal vitamin containing 400 IU vitamin D3 plus a vitamin D capsule containing 3,400 IU, both taken daily.	Prenatal vitamin containing 400 IU vitamin D3 plus a placebo capsule, both taken daily	12 weeks	Serum 25(OH)D	NA	NA
Wagner et al., 2013	Columbia, USA	Randomized, double-blinded study	12-16	>16	257	4000 IU	2000 IU	Till delivery	Serum 25(OH)D	Cord 25(OH)D	NA
Wei et al., 2017	South Carolina, USA	Randomized, double-blinded study	<16	16-45	301	400 IU, 2000 IU, and 4000 IU	No Comparison group	Till delivery	Maternal 25(OH)D	NA	Inadequacy: 50 nmol/L (20ng/mL), Adequacy: ≥50 nmol/L (≥20 ng/mL)
Zerofsky et al., 2016	California, USA	Randomized, double-blinded study	<20	>18	57	2000 IU	400 IU	Till delivery	25(OH)D concentration	Birth-weight, Apgar score	NA

Study ID	Country	Study Design	Trimester (weeks of gestation)	Mean age (years)	No. of participant	Intervention (With dose)	Control (With dose)	Duration	Maternal Outcomes	Neonatal Outcomes	Vitamin D cut offs and unit of measurement
OTHER REGIONS											
Grant et al., 2014	Auckland (latitude 36°S)	Randomized, double-blind, placebo-controlled multiarm parallel study	27	NA	260	Woman/infant pairs received a once-daily oral dose vitamin D3 1000 IU/400 IU, or vitamin D3 2000 IU/800 IU	Woman/infant pairs received a once-daily oral dose placebo/placebo	27 weeks' gestation to birth	Serum25(OH)D, Serum calcium	Cord blood 25(OH)D concentration, Serum25(OH)D of infants	Optimum threshold: ≥30 ng/mL
Rodda et al., 2015	Australia and New Zealand	Open label randomized study	12-16	≥18	78	2000 IU orally daily	NA	Until 28 weeks of gestation	Serum 25(OH)D	Cord 25(OH)D	Deficiency/insufficiency: <75 nmol/l

NA: Not Available, IUGR: Intrauterine Growth Retardation, hs-CRP: high sensitivity C-reactive protein, SBP: Systolic Blood Pressure, DBP: Diastolic Blood Pressure, FPG: Fasting Plasma Glucose, iPTH: Intact Parathyroid Hormone, SGA: Small for Gestation Age, ALP: Alkaline Phosphatase, HOMA-IR: Homeostatic model assessment Insulin Resistance, GDM: Gestational Diabetes Mellitus, IL: Interleukin, TNF: Tumor Necrosis Factor, BMC: Bone Mineral Content, BMD: Bone Mineral Density, GWG: Gestational Weight Gain, PIH: Pregnancy Induced Hypertension.

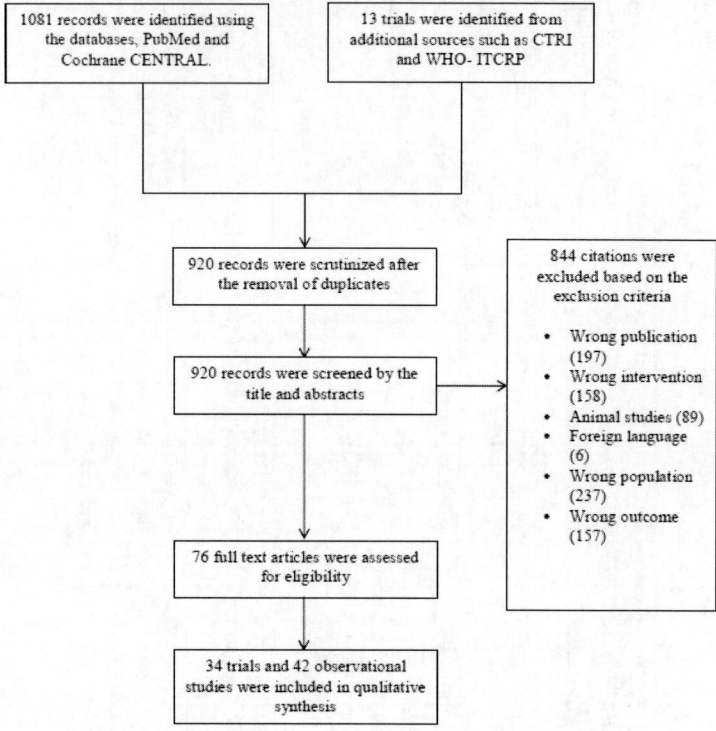

Figure 1. Study flow diagram.

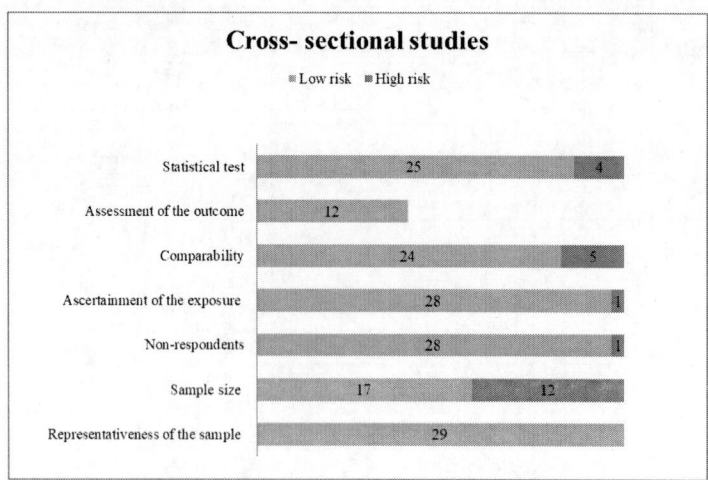

The numbers within the graph indicates the number of studies.

Figure 2. Risk of bias summary of cross- sectional studies.

3.1.2.2. Randomized Controlled Trials

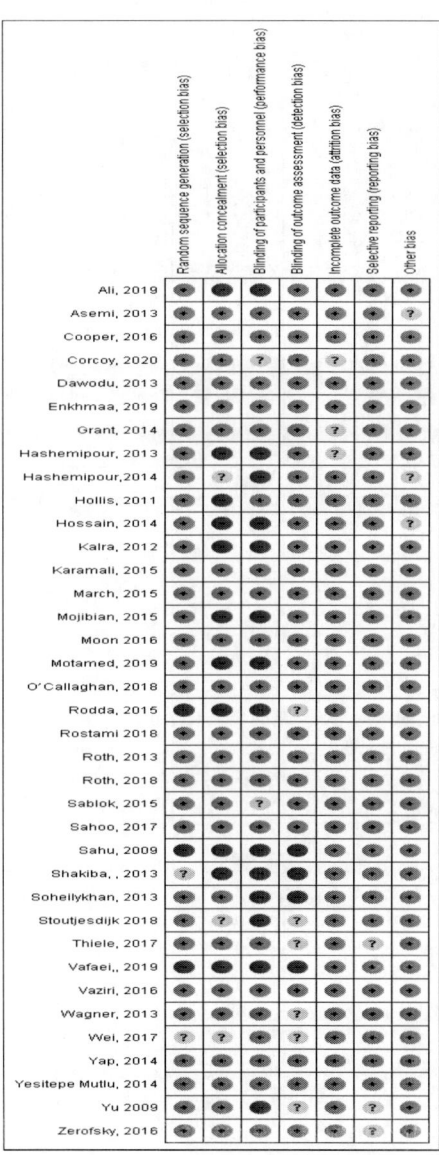

Figure 3. Risk of bias summary of clinical trials on Vitamin D supplementation.

Table 3. Risk of bias assessment of the included studies

Ali et al. (2019)

Bias	Author's judgment	Support for judgment
Random sequence generation (selection bias)	Low risk	Permuted block randomization was used for allocation into groups 1 and 2
Allocation concealment (selection bias)	High risk	Allocation concealment was not done
Blinding of participants and personnel (performance bias)	High risk	Blinding was not done since it is an open label study
Blinding of outcome assessment (detection bias)	Low risk	Objective measurement of outcomes
Incomplete outcome data (attrition bias)	Low risk	Only 4% of study participants were lost to follow-up
Selective reporting (reporting bias)	Low risk	All listed outcomes were reported
Other biases	Low risk	Authors have no other biases to declare

Asemi et al. (2013)

Bias	Author's judgment	Support for judgment
Random sequence generation (selection bias)	Low risk	Randomization was performed using computer generated random numbers
Allocation concealment (selection bias)	Low risk	Placebo was packed and coded identical to the intervention
Blinding of participants and personnel (performance bias)	Low risk	Study participants and investigators were blinded
Blinding of outcome assessment (detection bias)	Low risk	Outcomes measured using laboratory assays.
Incomplete outcome data (attrition bias)	Low risk	Attrition rate was 22% because of pregnancy complications.
Selective reporting (reporting bias)	Low risk	All outcomes were reported
Other biases	Unclear risk	Trial registration details were not stated

Cooper et al. (2016)

Bias	Author's judgment	Support for judgment
Random sequence generation (selection bias)	Low risk	Permuted block randomization was performed using a computer generated sequence
Allocation concealment (selection bias)	Low risk	The excipients in the placebo were matched to the intervention. They were blister packed in a similar way.
Blinding of participants and personnel (performance bias)	Low risk	The medications were supplied in coded envelopes
Blinding of outcome assessment (detection bias)	Low risk	Blinding was not required for outcome measurement
Incomplete outcome data (attrition bias)	Low risk	The authors had not reported any attrition
Selective reporting (reporting bias)	Low risk	All listed outcomes were reported
Other biases	Low risk	No other risk was identified

The Prevalence and Management of Vitamin D Deficiency ...

Bias	Author's judgment	Support for judgment
Corcoy et al. (2020)		
Random sequence generation (selection bias)	Low risk	Pre- stratification was done use a computer generated random number
Allocation concealment (selection bias)	Low risk	Sealed opaque envelopes were used for allocating the intervention and comparator
Blinding of participants and personnel (performance bias)	Unclear risk	Method of blinding was not stated
Blinding of outcome assessment (detection bias)	Low risk	Study personnel's involved in measurements were blinded
Incomplete outcome data (attrition bias)	Unclear risk	The exact attrition rate could not be calculated since the number of participants lost to follow up were varied in each of the measured time-points
Selective reporting (reporting bias)	Low risk	All outcomes stated were reported
Other biases	Low risk	No other biases were reported
Dawodu et al. (2013)		
Random sequence generation (selection bias)	Low risk	The participants were stratified into blocks to receive the intervention
Allocation concealment (selection bias)	Low risk	The study drugs were administered in same packaging and there were of same color and taste
Blinding of participants and personnel (performance bias)	Low risk	The participants, investigators and health-care providers were blinded
Blinding of outcome assessment (detection bias)	Low risk	Study personnel's involved in laboratory measurements were also blinded
Incomplete outcome data (attrition bias)	Low risk	15% attrition rate was reported due to unidentified reasons.
Selective reporting (reporting bias)	Low risk	All outcomes were reported
Other biases	Low risk	No other biases were reported
Enkhmaa et al. (2019)		
Random sequence generation (selection bias)	Low risk	Participants were stratified into blocks using randomly generated numbers
Allocation concealment (selection bias)	Low risk	The capsules used in the study were identical in appearance. Participant assignment numbers were provided in sealed envelopes
Blinding of participants and personnel (performance bias)	Low risk	Participants, clinicians and investigators were blinded
Blinding of outcome assessment (detection bias)	Low risk	Blinding of laboratory technicians were unnecessary
Incomplete outcome data (attrition bias)	Low risk	The authors had not reported any attrition due to the intervention
Selective reporting (reporting bias)	Low risk	All outcomes listed were reported
Other biases		No other biases were identified

Table 3. (Continued)

Grant et al. (2014)		
Bias	Author's judgment	Support for judgment
Random sequence generation (selection bias)	Low risk	Computer generated randomization list was used
Allocation concealment (selection bias)	Low risk	The study medications are identical in their taste, appearance, consistency and labeling
Blinding of participants and personnel (performance bias)	Low risk	The interventions were coded to ensure blinding of study participants and staff
Blinding of outcome assessment (detection bias)	Low risk	Blinding was not necessary was laboratory measurements
Incomplete outcome data (attrition bias)	Unclear risk	Only 77% of cord blood samples were retained. The reason for withdrawal was not stated clearly.
Selective reporting (reporting bias)	Low risk	All outcomes were reported
Other biases	Low risk	No other biases were identified
Hashemipour et al. (2013)		
Random sequence generation (selection bias)	Low risk	Computer generated random numbers were used for randomization
Allocation concealment (selection bias)	High risk	No information on allocation concealment was provided
Blinding of participants and personnel (performance bias)	High risk	Blinding was not done since it was an open labeled trial
Blinding of outcome assessment (detection bias)	Low risk	Blinding is not required for laboratory assessments
Incomplete outcome data (attrition bias)	Unclear risk	Though only 68% of the participants were retained in the study, the loss to follow up was not stated to be due to adverse effects of the intervention
Selective reporting (reporting bias)	Low risk	All outcomes were measured and reported
Other biases	Low risk	No other biases were detected
Hashemipour et al. (2014)		
Random sequence generation (selection bias)	Low risk	Randomization was done using computer generated numbers
Allocation concealment (selection bias)	Unclear risk	Though the authors gad stated allocation concealment, the method used for the same was not given
Blinding of participants and personnel (performance bias)	High risk	Blinding was not done since it was an open label trial
Blinding of outcome assessment (detection bias)	Low risk	Blinding of laboratory personnel was not required.
Incomplete outcome data (attrition bias)	Low risk	There was no loss of participants due to the intervention
Selective reporting (reporting bias)	Low risk	

Bias	Author's judgment	Support for judgment
	Unclear risk	All outcomes listed were measured and reported
Other biases		Compliance of the participants to the study medications was not reported
Hollis et al. (2011)		
Random sequence generation (selection bias)	Low risk	Participants were randomly stratified into blocks based on their ethnic groups
Allocation concealment (selection bias)	High risk	No information on the allocation concealment was provided
Blinding of participants and personnel (performance bias)	Low risk	Participants and investigators were blinded
Blinding of outcome assessment (detection bias)	Low risk	Obstetricians involved in monitoring patient health status were blinded
Incomplete outcome data (attrition bias)	Low risk	There was no significant loss to follow up among treatment groups
Selective reporting (reporting bias)	Low risk	All outcomes listed were reported
Other biases	Low risk	No other biases were identified
Hossain et al. (2014)		
Random sequence generation (selection bias)	Low risk	Sequential randomization technique was used
Allocation concealment (selection bias)	High risk	Allocation concealment was not performed
Blinding of participants and personnel (performance bias)	High risk	Study participants and investigators were not blinded since it is an open label trial
Blinding of outcome assessment (detection bias)	Low risk	Blinding was not necessary
Incomplete outcome data (attrition bias)	Low risk	Attrition rate was not significant
Selective reporting (reporting bias)	Low risk	All outcomes listed were reported
Other biases	High risk	The control arm was not provided with a routine dose of vitamin D supplementation
Kalra et al. (2012)		
Random sequence generation (selection bias)	Low risk	Random allocation number was used for randomization
Allocation concealment (selection bias)	High risk	Allocation concealment was not done
Blinding of participants and personnel (performance bias)	High risk	Participants and personnel's were not blinded
Blinding of outcome assessment (detection bias)	Low risk	Outcomes were measured objectively
Incomplete outcome data (attrition bias)	Low risk	Though 32% of the subjects were lost to follow up, It was not due to the adverse effect of the intervention
Selective reporting (reporting bias)	Low risk	All outcomes listed were reported
Other biases	Low risk	No other biases were found

Table 3. (Continued)

Karamali et al. (2015)		
Bias	Author's judgment	Support for judgment
Random sequence generation (selection bias)	Low risk	Participants were randomized using a computer generated sequence
Allocation concealment (selection bias)	Low risk	Placebo and intervention were similar in appearance
Blinding of participants and personnel (performance bias)	Low risk	The trial medications were administered in numbered bottles and blinded from participants and researchers. Blinding was performed until the completion of analysis
Blinding of outcome assessment (detection bias)	Low risk	All included participants had completed the study
Incomplete outcome data (attrition bias)	Low risk	All outcomes were reported
Selective reporting (reporting bias)	Low risk	No other biases were identified
Other biases	Low risk	
March et al. (2015)		
Random sequence generation (selection bias)	Low risk	Participants were randomly allocated by block randomization; based on ethnicity
Allocation concealment (selection bias)	Low risk	The supplements were identical in appearance
Blinding of participants and personnel (performance bias)	Low risk	All supplements were coded to ensure blinding
Blinding of outcome assessment (detection bias)	Low risk	Blinding was not necessary since external validation was used for analyses
Incomplete outcome data (attrition bias)	Low risk	The study authors maintained a retention rate of 76%
Selective reporting (reporting bias)	Low risk	All outcomes listed were reported
Other biases	Low risk	No other biases were identified
Mojibian et al. (2015)		
Random sequence generation (selection bias)	Low risk	The participants were randomly allocated using a computer generated sequence
Allocation concealment (selection bias)	High risk	The trial medications were not concealed at the time of administration
Blinding of participants and personnel (performance bias)	High risk	Participants and researchers were not blinded
Blinding of outcome assessment (detection bias)	Low risk	Outcomes were assessed using laboratory measurement
Incomplete outcome data (attrition bias)	Low risk	Only 6% of the participants had discontinued the trial medications
Selective reporting (reporting bias)	Low risk	All outcomes were reported
Other biases	Low risk	No other biases were identified

Moon et al. (2016)		
Bias	Author's judgment	Support for judgment
Random sequence generation (selection bias)	Low risk	Permuted block randomization using a computer generated sequence was used
Allocation concealment (selection bias)	Low risk	The placebo was matched to the intervention
Blinding of participants and personnel (performance bias)	Low risk	Both participants and researchers were masked from the treatment
Blinding of outcome assessment (detection bias)	Low risk	Outcomes were assessed using laboratory measurement
Incomplete outcome data (attrition bias)	Low risk	Only 6% of the participants had discontinued the trial medications
Selective reporting (reporting bias)	Low risk	All outcomes were reported
Other biases		No other biases were identified
Motamed et al. (2019)		
Random sequence generation (selection bias)	Low risk	Subjects were randomized into two groups using block randomization
Allocation concealment (selection bias)	High risk	Allocation concealment was not performed
Blinding of participants and personnel (performance bias)	High risk	Being an Open labeled trial, blinding was not performed
Blinding of outcome assessment (detection bias)	Low risk	Outcomes were laboratory measurements
Incomplete outcome data (attrition bias)	Low risk	The authors did not report any significant attrition
Selective reporting (reporting bias)	Low risk	All outcomes were reported
Other biases	Low risk	No other biases were identified
O'Callaghan et al. (2018)		
Random sequence generation (selection bias)	Low risk	Computer generated randomization list was prepared by a scientist inert to study analysis
Allocation concealment (selection bias)	Low risk	The appearance, packaging and taste of both placebo and intervention were identical
Blinding of participants and personnel (performance bias)	Low risk	Study participants and investigators were blinded
Blinding of outcome assessment (detection bias)	Low risk	Laboratory generated results, hence blinding was not required
Incomplete outcome data (attrition bias)	Low risk	84% of the participants were retained after administration of the intervention. Loss to follow up was due to adverse pregnancy outcomes and not due to the intervention
Selective reporting (reporting bias)	Low risk	All outcomes listed in the protocol were measured and reported
Other biases	Low risk	No other bias was reported

Table 3. (Continued)

Rodda et al. (2015)		
Bias	Author's judgment	Support for judgment
Random sequence generation (selection bias)	High risk	No randomization performed
Allocation concealment (selection bias)	High risk	Not done
Blinding of participants and personnel (performance bias)	High risk	Open label study
Blinding of outcome assessment (detection bias)	Unclear risk	Not mentioned
Incomplete outcome data (attrition bias)	Low risk	Not much attrition
Selective reporting (reporting bias)	Low risk	All the data were analyzed
Other biases	Low risk	No other bias was reported
Rostami et al. (2018)		
Random sequence generation (selection bias)	Low risk	Randomization was performed in blocks of four using a computer-generated list
Allocation concealment (selection bias)	Low risk	Physicians, who participated in various phases of the study, were blinded to grouping of women
Blinding of participants and personnel (performance bias)	Low risk	
Blinding of outcome assessment (detection bias)	Low risk	Health care workers who determined pregnancy outcomes were blinded to treatment allocation
Incomplete outcome data (attrition bias)	Low risk	Assessor was blinded
Selective reporting (reporting bias)	Low risk	Not much of attrition rate
Other biases		All the outcome measures are listed
		No other bias was reported
Roth et al. (2013)		
Random sequence generation (selection bias)	Low risk	Assignment was based on a compute regenerated randomization list, with the block size of 4 and 8.
Allocation concealment (selection bias)	Low risk	The allocation sequences was prepared who was not part of the study
Blinding of participants and personnel (performance bias)	Low risk	Participants and research staff (including lab personnel) were blinded to allocation.
Blinding of outcome assessment (detection bias)	Low risk	The outcome assessor was blinded
Incomplete outcome data (attrition bias)	Low risk	Lost to follow was lo
Selective reporting (reporting bias)	Low risk	All the data in the study was reported
Other biases	Low risk	No other bias was reported
Roth et al. (2018)		
Random sequence generation (selection bias)	Low risk	A computer-generated, simple randomization scheme was created independently by the trial statistician.
Allocation concealment (selection bias)	Low risk	
Blinding of participants and personnel (performance bias)	Low risk	
	Low risk	

Bias	Author's judgment	Support for judgment
Blinding of outcome assessment (detection bias)	Low risk	Concealment of trial-group assignments was ensured and its use was pre-labeled and sequentially numbered.
Incomplete outcome data (attrition bias)	Low risk	The Participants and the study personnel were blinded
Selective reporting (reporting bias)		Yes, the assessor was blinded
Other biases		The data was analyzed for all the participants as per intent to treat
		All the reported outcomes were analyzed.
		No other bias was reported
Sablok et al. (2015)		
Random sequence generation (selection bias)	Low risk	Computer generated random table was generated
Allocation concealment (selection bias)	Low risk	Concealment of the group was done
Blinding of participants and personnel (performance bias)	Unclear risk	No details were provided
Blinding of outcome assessment (detection bias)	Low risk	The assessor was blinded
Incomplete outcome data (attrition bias)	Low risk	Attrition rate was low
Selective reporting (reporting bias)	Low risk	All the outcome data was reported
Other biases	Low risk	No other biases
Sahoo et al. (2017)		
Random sequence generation (selection bias)	Low risk	Randomization was done by a computer-generated sequence in a randomly permuted blocks of hundred
Allocation concealment (selection bias)	Low risk	All the medications were dispensed in sequentially numbered, identical, opaque, sealed packs (carrying the name of the participant) by a research assistant, who was blinded to intervention
Blinding of participants and personnel (performance bias)	Unclear risk	Blinding was followed
Blinding of outcome assessment (detection bias)	Low risk	Yes, the assessor was blinded
Incomplete outcome data (attrition bias)	Low risk	The attrition rate was low
Selective reporting (reporting bias)	Low risk	All outcomes are reported
Other biases	Low risk	No other biases
Sahu et al. (2009)		
Random sequence generation (selection bias)	High risk	Randomization was abandoned, Because it was unethical to continue with a group not receiving any cholecalciferol.
Allocation concealment (selection bias)	High risk	No details provided
Blinding of participants and personnel (performance bias)	High risk	Not blinded
Blinding of outcome assessment (detection bias)	High risk	Not mentioned
	Low risk	Lost to follow up was not present
	Low risk	
	Low risk	

Table 3. (Continued)

Bias	Author's judgment	Support for judgment
Incomplete outcome data (attrition bias) Selective reporting (reporting bias) Other biases		Outcome measure were reported No other biases were identified
Shakiba et al. (2013)		
Random sequence generation (selection bias) Allocation concealment (selection bias) Blinding of participants and personnel (performance bias) Blinding of outcome assessment (detection bias) Incomplete outcome data (attrition bias) Selective reporting (reporting bias) Other biases	Unclear risk High risk High risk High risk Low risk Low risk Low risk	The participants were randomly recruited, and the details of the randomization are not mentioned Not mentioned Not mentioned The details of the assessor blinded not mentioned Analysis of the data was done on all outcome measures All the outcome measure was accounted in the analysis No other biases were identified
Soheilykhan et al. (2013)		
Random sequence generation (selection bias) Allocation concealment (selection bias) Blinding of participants and personnel (performance bias) Blinding of outcome assessment (detection bias) Incomplete outcome data (attrition bias) Selective reporting (reporting bias) Other biases	Low risk Low risk High risk High risk Low risk Low risk Low risk	Computer-generated random number lists were drawn up by an independent researcher Allocation concealment was maintained Pregnant women and researchers were not blinded to treatment assignment Assessor was not blinded Dropout rate was low All the data was reported No other biases
Stoutjesdijk et al. (2013)		
Random sequence generation (selection bias) Allocation concealment (selection bias) Blinding of participants and personnel (performance bias) Blinding of outcome assessment (detection bias) Incomplete outcome data (attrition bias) Selective reporting (reporting bias) Other biases	Low risk Unclear risk High risk Unclear risk Low risk Low risk Low risk	Block randomization method was used Not mentioned Not blinded Not mentioned Less dropout rates All data was analyzed as stated No other biases were identified

Thiele et al. (2017)		
Bias	Author's judgment	Support for judgment
Random sequence generation (selection bias)	Low risk	A random sequence generator was used for group assignment corresponding to the participant numbers in a 1:1 ratio
Allocation concealment (selection bias)	Low risk	The random sequence was generated independently from the research team.
Blinding of participants and personnel (performance bias)	Low risk	Blinding of the intervention was maintained at the level of participants, the data collector, and the data analyst until completion of all data collection.
Blinding of outcome assessment	Unclear risk	
	Low risk	
(detection bias)	Unclear risk	Not mentioned
Incomplete outcome data (attrition bias)		Not much of dropout rate
Selective reporting (reporting bias)	Low risk	All outcome measure were reported and analyzed
Other biases		No other biases were identified
Vafaei et al. (2019)		
Random sequence generation (selection bias)	High risk	Randomization was not done
	High risk	Not mentioned
Allocation concealment (selection bias)	High risk	Not mentioned
Blinding of participants and personnel (performance bias)		Not mentioned
	High risk	Attrition rate was low
Blinding of outcome assessment	Low risk	All outcomes were measured
(detection bias)	Low risk	No other biases were identified
Incomplete outcome data (attrition bias)	Low risk	
Selective reporting (reporting bias)		
Other biases		
Vaziri et al. (2016)		
Random sequence generation (selection bias)	Low risk	Block Randomization method was used
	Low risk	Was performed
Allocation concealment (selection bias)	Low risk	Participants and the study personnel were blinded
Blinding of participants and personnel (performance bias)	Low risk	The assessor was blinded
Blinding of outcome assessment (detection bias)	Low risk	127 study participants completed the study, thus attrition rate was within the range
Incomplete outcome data (attrition bias)	Low risk	All outcomes were reported
Selective reporting (reporting bias)	Low risk	No other biases were identified
Other biases		
Wagner et al. (2013)		
Random sequence generation (selection bias)	Low risk	Randomization lists were generated by computer prior to the start of the study.
Allocation concealment (selection bias)	Low risk	Randomization assignment was blinded to all participants and to the investigators except for the study biostatistician.

Table 3. (Continued)

Bias	Author's judgment	Support for judgment
Blinding of participants and personnel (performance bias)	Low risk	Both study personnel and participants were blinded
Blinding of outcome assessment (detection bias)	Unclear risk	Not mentioned
Incomplete outcome data (attrition bias)	Low risk	Low lost to follow up rate
Selective reporting (reporting bias)	Low risk	All the outcome measure was measured as stated
Other biases	Low risk	No other biases were identified
Wei et al. (2017)		
Random sequence generation (selection bias)	Unclear risk	Not mentioned
Allocation concealment (selection bias)	Unclear risk	Not mentioned
Blinding of participants and personnel (performance bias)	Low risk	Double blind study
Blinding of outcome assessment (detection bias)	Unclear risk	Not mentioned
Incomplete outcome data (attrition bias)	Low risk	Low dropouts
Selective reporting (reporting bias)	Low risk	All the mentioned outcome data was analyzed
Other biases	Low risk	No other biases were identified
Yap et al. (2014)		
Random sequence generation (selection bias)	Low risk	Permuted block size of six and sequential assignment was performed
Allocation concealment (selection bias)	Low risk	Allocation concealment was maintained
Blinding of participants and personnel (performance bias)	Low risk	Study investigators and participants were blinded to the intervention allocated.
Blinding of outcome assessment (detection bias)	Low risk	Assessor was blinded
Incomplete outcome data (attrition bias)	Low risk	Dropout rate was low
Selective reporting (reporting bias)	Low risk	All the data were analyzed
Other biases	Low risk	No other biases were identified
Yesitepe Mutlu et al. (2014)		
Random sequence generation (selection bias)	Low risk	Randomization was performed
Allocation concealment (selection bias)	Low risk	Was performed
Blinding of participants and personnel (performance bias)	Low risk	The study personnel and participants were blinded
Blinding of outcome assessment (detection bias)	Low risk	The assessor was blinded
Incomplete outcome data (attrition bias)	Low risk	The attrition rate was low
Selective reporting (reporting bias)	Low risk	All the stated outcome data were assessed
Other biases	Low risk	No other biases were identified

Bias	Author's judgment	Support for judgment
Yu et al. (2009)		
Random sequence generation (selection bias)	Low risk	Computer generated random number lists were drawn
Allocation concealment (selection bias)	Low risk	Allocation concealment was maintained
Blinding of participants and personnel (performance bias)	High risk	All study personnel and participants were not blinded to treatment assignment
Blinding of outcome assessment (detection bias)	Unclear risk	Not mentioned
Incomplete outcome data (attrition bias)	Low risk	Exclusion from analysis data were zero thus no attrition bias found
Selective reporting (reporting bias)	Unclear risk	Not mentioned
Other biases	Low risk	No other biases were identified
Zerofsky et al. (2016)		
Random sequence generation (selection bias)	Low risk	Block-randomized list was generated in sequential order as they participants were enrolled.
Allocation concealment (selection bias)	Low risk	Allocation concealment was maintained
Blinding of participants and personnel (performance bias)	Low risk	Study staff and participants were blinded to the treatment group for the duration of the study.
Blinding of outcome assessment (detection bias)	Unclear risk	For study participants at UCDMC, the electronic medical record was used to collect data on the results
Incomplete outcome data (attrition bias)	Low risk	The drop rate was low
Selective reporting (reporting bias)	Unclear risk	All the outcome measure was analyzed as stated
Other biases	Low risk	No other biases were identified

The quality of 37 randomized controlled trials was assessed. The bias assessment is summarized in Figure 3 and author judgments are stated in Table 3. Three trials (Rodda 2015, Sahu 2009, and Vafaei 2019) [77, 79, 95] indicated a 'high risk' for selection bias since the randomization technique was not stated by the authors. Improper concealment of treatment allocation from the study participants led to 'high risk' in 11 studies. The study participants and personnel's were not blinded in 11 trials (Ali 2019 [21], Hashemipour 2013, Hashemipour 2014 [66], Hossain 2014 [67], Kalra 2012 [68], Mojibian 2015 [70], Motamed 2019 [71], Rodda 2015 [95], Sahoo 2017 [76], Stoutjesdijk 2018 [86], and Yu 2009 [87]) and the method of blinding was not specified in 5 trials (Corcoy 2020 [83], Sablok 2015

[75], Sahu 2009 [77], Vafaie 2019 [79] and Shakiba 2013 [78]). Blinding of outcome assessors was not required as most them were measured objectively. Though the attrition rate varied between studies, there was not significant loss to follow up due to adverse effects of Vitamin D supplementation. There was a 'high risk' of ethical concerns associated with Hossain 2014 since the treatment was not balanced between both the arms. Vitamin D deficiency in the untreated arm increased the risk of pre-eclampsia, gestational hypertension, and small foe gestational age.

3.2. Outcomes

3.2.1. Prevalence of Vitamin D Deficiency

Proportion Meta- analysis was conducted by computing the number of cases of Vitamin D deficiency and total cases. Random effect modeling was used due to the increase in heterogeneity. The proportion of Vitamin D deficiency during pregnancy was analyzed to be 69.98%, across the globe. The pooled prevalence was then categorized based on geographical regions. The prevalence was found to be 82.4% (95% CI 76.01 to 88.10) for the studies conducted in Asian population. The model was statistically significant at $p< 0.001$ and a high heterogeneity of 96.71%. The European studies showed a prevalence of 51.46% (95% CI 38.46 to 64.36) of Vitamin D deficiency in a sample size of 5491 pregnant women. The I^2 value was found to be 98.81%, which was highly significant at $p < 0.0001$. Data published in studies across other parts of the world indicated a proportion of 61.9% (95% CI 37.13 to 83.74). The heterogeneity was high with an I^2 of 99.5%. The results of the proportion Meta- analysis is summarized in Table 4.

3.2.2. Maternal Outcomes

3.2.2.1. Maternal 25 (OH) D Levels (nmol/L)

At the time of analysis, the included trials were broadly categorized as placebo- controlled trials and Vitamin D dose comparison studies. 14

placebo- controlled trials with a total sample size of 3,073 participants were analyzed. Maternal 25 (OH) D levels had improved significantly in the Vitamin D supplemented group (MD 31.04, 95% CI 21.33 to 40.75). Random effect modeling was used since the level of heterogeneity was extremely high ($I^2 = 98\%$). The forest plot on maternal 25 (OH) D levels in depicted in Figure 4. Sub- group analysis was conducted based on dose, duration of Vitamin D supplementation, sample size, and region. Though the overall effect showed significant improvement in maternal vitamin D levels in all subgroups, the I^2 value was 98% (Figure 5, 6, 7, 8). Further subgroup analyses were stopped due to unimproved heterogeneity. A total of 13 trials on dose comparison of Vitamin D were included for analyses. The doses were classified into two groups (<2000IU Vitamin D vs. ≥2000IU Vitamin D). This range was selected based on the maximum dose of Vitamin D supplementation approved for use in pregnant women by various treatment guidelines. The mean and standard deviation of multi-arm studies were combined to meet the above criteria. The pooled effect of 25 (OH) D levels were significantly high when administered with ≥2000IU Vitamin D (MD -30.16, 95% CI -37.83 to -22.49) at p < 0.00001 ($I^2 = 93\%$). The forest plot is depicted in Figure 9. The results of sub- group analyses are summarized in Table 5.

Study or Subgroup	Vitamin D Mean	SD	Total	Placebo Mean	SD	Total	Weight	Mean Difference IV, Random, 95% CI
Asemi, 2013	53.75	4.5	24	33.25	2.75	24	7.7%	20.50 [18.39, 22.61]
Cooper, 2016	67.8	22.1	425	43.3	22.3	440	7.6%	24.50 [21.54, 27.46]
Corcoy, 2020	122.9	38.8	79	84.5	39.8	75	6.8%	38.40 [25.98, 50.82]
Grant, 2014	98.99	12.82	150	51.2	12.99	78	7.6%	47.79 [44.25, 51.33]
Kalra, 2012	46.62	19.77	96	43.25	15.08	48	7.5%	3.37 [-2.45, 9.19]
Karamali, 2015	87.14	5.89	30	43.36	10.08	30	7.6%	43.78 [39.60, 47.96]
Moon 2016	67.7	21.3	407	43.1	22.5	422	7.6%	24.60 [21.62, 27.58]
O'Callaghan, 2018	98.49	26.09	81	71.4	24.3	40	7.2%	27.09 [17.66, 36.52]
Rodda, 2015	71	43.04	22	36	30.08	23	5.5%	35.00 [13.22, 56.78]
Roth, 2013	134.4	30.7	80	38.4	18.1	80	7.3%	96.00 [88.19, 103.81]
Sablok, 2015	80	51.53	108	46.11	74.21	57	5.6%	33.89 [12.31, 55.47]
Sahoo, 2017	55.28	21.1	36	24.5	17.3	16	7.0%	30.78 [19.85, 41.71]
Sahu, 2009	30.9	23.3	35	23.8	3.85	14	7.3%	7.10 [-0.88, 15.08]
Vaziri, 2016	17.46	10.09	78	12.07	5.98	75	7.6%	5.39 [2.77, 8.01]
Total (95% CI)			1651			1422	100.0%	31.04 [21.33, 40.75]

Heterogeneity: Tau² = 319.41; Chi² = 865.71, df = 13 (P < 0.00001); I² = 98%
Test for overall effect: Z = 6.26 (P < 0.00001)

Figure 4. Forest plot of Maternal 25 (OH) D levels [Vitamin D Vs Placebo].

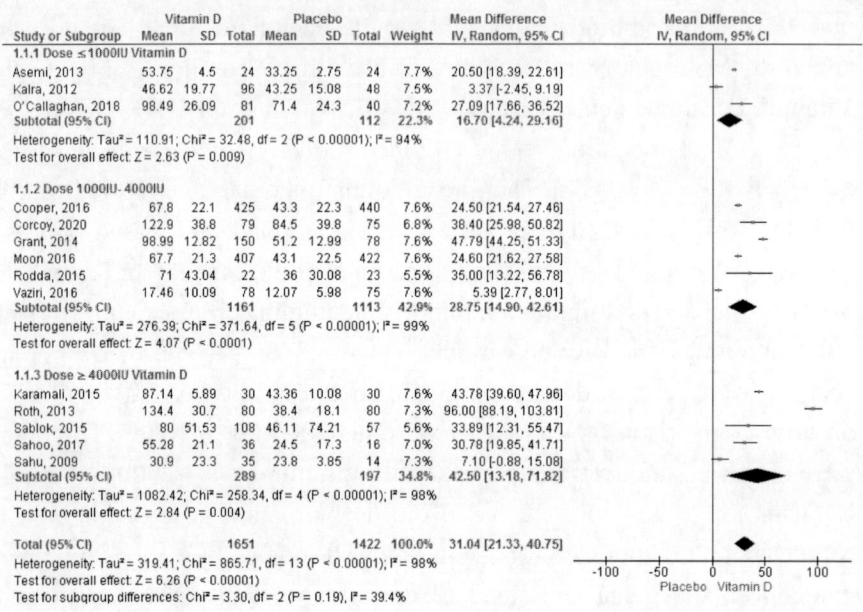

Figure 5. Sub-group analysis of maternal 25(OH) D levels based on dose.

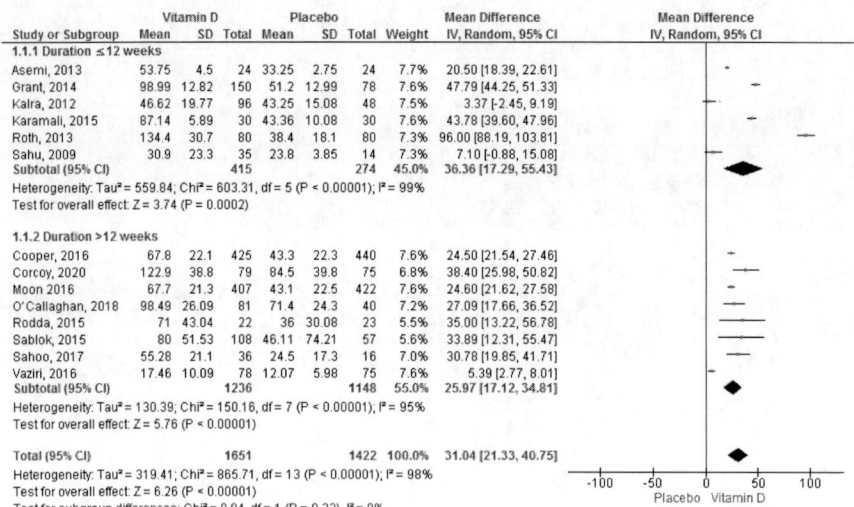

Figure 6. Sub-group analysis of maternal 25(OH) D levels based on treatment duration.

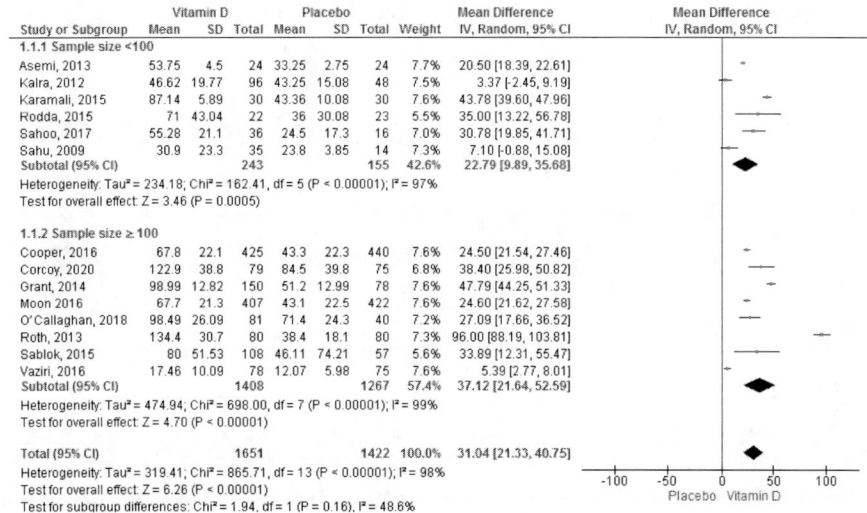

Figure 7. Sub- group analysis of maternal 25(OH) D levels based on sample size.

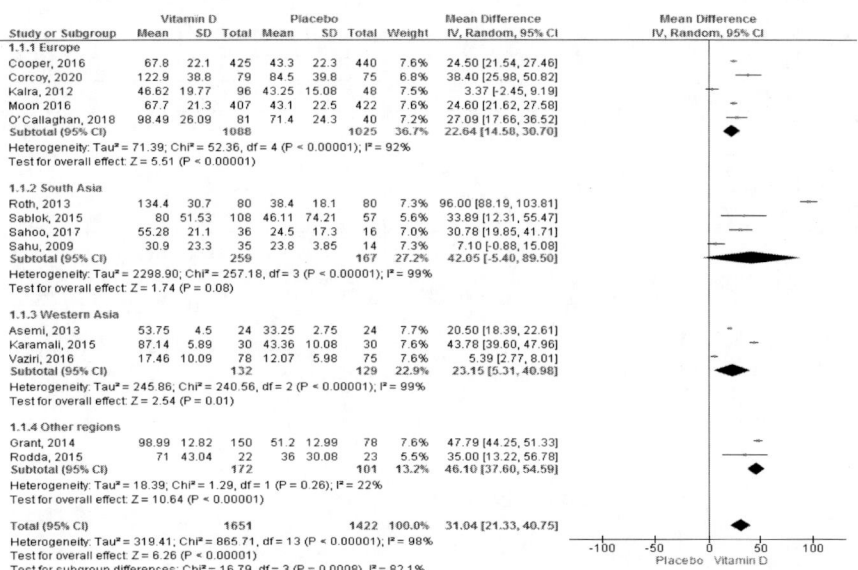

Figure 8. Sub- group analysis of maternal 25(OH) D levels based on region

Table 4. Results of meta- proportion analysis on the prevalence of Vitamin D deficiency in pregnancy

Meta-proportion analysis	Number of studies	Number of participants	Proportion (%)	95% CI	Test for heterogeneity	
					I^2 (%)	P value
Overall prevalence						
(i) Fixed effect	42	14466	67.08	66.31 to 67.84	99.21	<0.0001
(ii) Random effect			69.98	61.07 to 78.18		
Asia						
(i) Fixed effect	20	5338	83.57	82.55 to 84.55	96.71	<0.0001
(ii) Random effect			82.47	76.01 to 88.10		
Europe						
(i) Fixed effect	13	5491	44.84	43.52 to 46.17	98.81	<0.0001
(ii) Random effect			51.46	38.46 to 64.36		
Other regions of the world						
(i) Fixed effect	9	3637	72.25	70.77 to 73.70	99.55	<0.0001
(ii) Random effect			61.90	37.13 to 83.74		

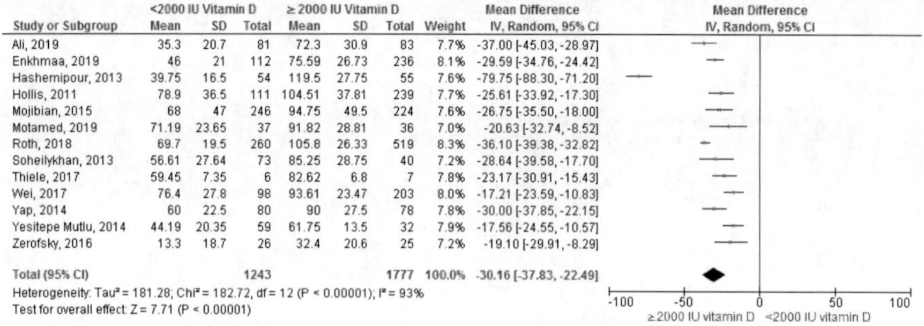

Figure 9. Forest plot on maternal 25(OH) D levels [High dose Vs Low dose].

Table 5. Results of sub-group analysis

Subgroup Analysis	Number of studies	Number of participants Vitamin D	Number of participants Placebo	Heterogeneity I^2	Heterogeneity P value	MD (95% CI)	P Value	Subgroup difference I^2	Subgroup difference P value
1. Maternal Serum 25(OH)D (nmol/L)									
(i) Vitamin D dosing								39.4%	0.19
a. ≤1000IU Vitamin D	3	203	112	94%	<0.00001	16.70(4.24, 29.16)	0.009		
b. 1000-4000 IU Vitamin D	6	1161	1113	99%	<0.00001	28.75(14.90, 42.61)	<0.00001		
c. ≥4000 IU Vitamin D	5	289	197	98%	<0.00001	42.50(13.18, 71.82)	0.004		
(ii) Treatment duration								0%	0.33
a. ≤12 weeks	6	415	274	99%	<0.00001	36.36(17.29, 55.43)	0.0002		
b. >12 weeks	8	1236	1148	95%	<0.00001	25.97(17.12, 34.81)	<0.00001		
(iii) Sample size								48.6%	0.16
a. <100	6	243	115	97%	<0.00001	22.79(9.89, 35.68)	0.0005		
b. ≥100	8	1651	1422	99%	<0.00001	37.12(21.54, 52.59)	<0.00001		
(iv) Geographical region								82.1%	0.0008
a. Europe	5	1088	1025	92%	<0.00001	22.64(14.58,30.70)	<0.00001		
b. South Asia	4	259	167	99%	<0.00001	42.05(-5.40,89.50)	0.08		
c. Western Asia	3	132	129	99%	<0.00001	23.15(5.31, 40.98)	0.01		
d. Others	2	172	101	98%	<0.00001	46.10(37.60,54.59)	<0.00001		
2. Cord 25(OH)D (nmol/L)									
(i) Treatment duration								54.8%	0.14
a. ≤12 weeks	4	1103	424	100%	<0.00001	31.15 (13.57, 48.74)	0.0005		
b. >12 weeks	8	809	562	88%	<0.00001	17.32 (12.39, 22.24)	<0.00001		
(ii) Sample size								0%	0.87
a. <100	4	185	114	74%	0.009	24.29 (13.69, 34.89)	<0.00001		
b. ≥100	8	1727	872	100%	<0.00001	22.97 (10.54, 35.40)	0.0003		

3.2.2.2. Serum Calcium (mmol/L) and Parathyroid Hormone (pmol/L) Levels

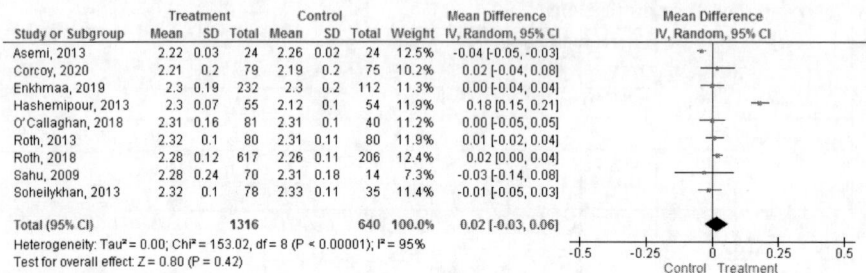

Figure 10. Forest plot on maternal serum calcium levels.

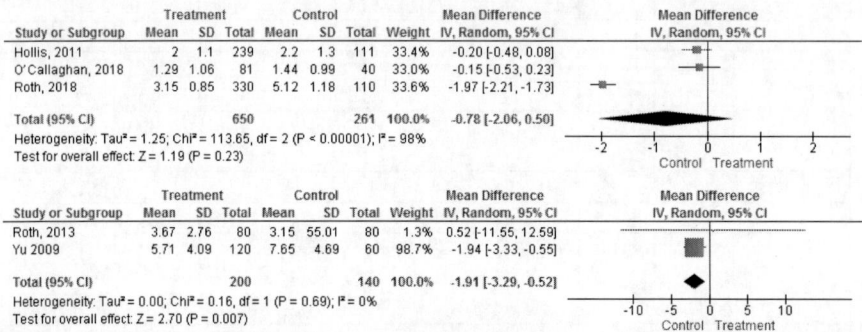

Figure 11. Forest plot on maternal iPTH and PTH levels.

Vitamin D induced hypercalcemia was assessed from the results of 9 studies. Only one study by Hashemipour et al. (2014) [66] had shown a significant incidence of hypercalcemia among pregnant women supplemented with a weekly dose of 50,000IU Vitamin D. However, the overall effect showed indifference in serum calcium elevation among treatment and control groups (MD 0.02, 95% CI -0.03 to 0.06, I^2 95%). The forest plot of maternal calcium levels is depicted in Figure 10. Three studies had reported parathyroid hormone levels, while two trials had reported intact parathyroid hormone levels. The parathyroid hormone levels were equally distributed in both the groups (MD -0.78, 95% CI -2.06 to 0.50 I^2 95%). The intact parathyroid hormone level was significantly elevated in the control group than Vitamin D supplemented group (MD -1.91, 95% CI -3.29 to -0.52, I^2 0%). The forest plot is depicted in Figure 11.

3.2.2.3. Pre- Eclampsia

The risk of vitamin D supplementation in the development of pre- eclampsia was estimated by pooling the results of 6 studies. The overall effect indicated indifference in the risk of pre- eclampsia in treatment and control group. The control group consisted of subjects administered with placebo or low dose Vitamin D. 48 participants out of 1070, from both treatment and control groups had developed pre- eclampsia (RR 0.77, 95% CI 0.34 to 1.76). There was only moderate level of heterogeneity (I^2 = 38%) within the included studies (Figure 12). Ali et al. reported extremely high incidence of pre- eclampsia in the regular dose (400IU) group.

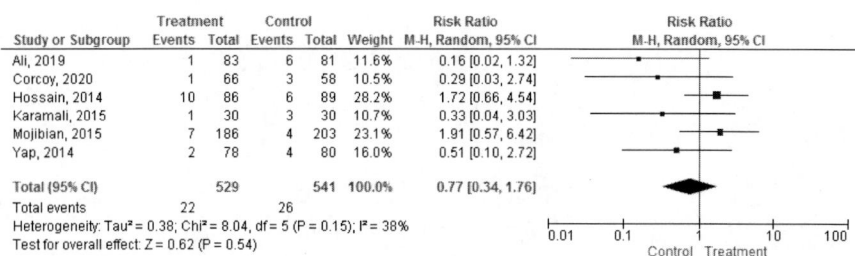

Figure 12. Forest plot on risk of pre- eclampsia with Vitamin D supplementation.

3.2.2.4. Gestational Diabetes Mellitus

In total, 5 studies with 1096 participants were included in the analysis: Ali 2019 [21]; Corcoy 2020 [83]; Hossain 2014 [67]; Mojibian 2015 [70]; Yap 2014 [96]. The result suggests that there is no difference in the development of gestational diabetes between treatment and control groups (RR 0.73, 95% CI 0.51 to 1.06). A total of 55 out of 1096 participants had developed gestational diabetes mellitus in the treatment group. The level of heterogeneity was 19% between the included studies (Figure 13).

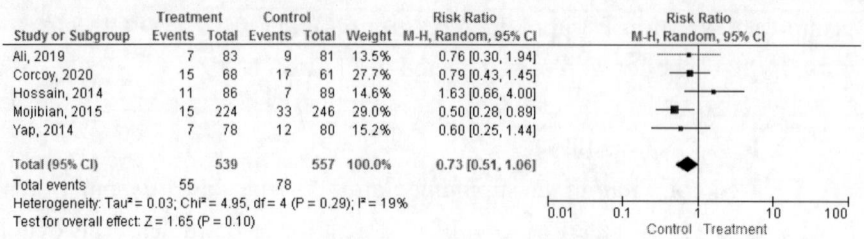

Figure 13. Forest plot on risk of gestational diabetes mellitus with Vitamin D supplementation.

3.2.2.5. Others

Certain studies had reported additional maternal outcomes such as bone mineral content, weight gain, inflammatory biomarkers etc. Brief descriptions of the additional outcomes are listed in Table 6. The outcomes were varied between the studies which could be a result of variation in trial methodology.

Table 6. Additional maternal and neonatal outcomes

Outcomes	Study results
IUGR	Ali (2019) showed a greater risk in the group treated with a routine dose (400IU) of vitamin D.
Neonatal BMC	Cooper (2016) reported no substantial improvement
hs- CRP	Asemi (2013)- negative correlation with vitamin D supplementation, Motamed (2019)- Positive correlation, Karamali (2015)- No effect
GWG	Hashemipour (2014), Moon (2016)- significant weight gain, Motamed (2019) and Corcoy (2020)- no change
Pro- inflammatory mediators	Motamed (2019)- increased circulation in mothers and infants supplemented with 2000 IU vitamin D.
Insulin resistance pattern	Karamali (2015)- Significant effect, Corcoy (2020)- no change
Blood pressure	Asemi (2013)- Decreased
Lipid profile	Karamali (2015)- Increase in high density lipoprotein

IUGR: Intrauterine growth retardation, BMC: Bone Mineral Content, hs- CRP: high sensitivity C reactive protein, GWG: Gestational weight gain.

3.2.3. Neonatal Outcomes

3.2.3.1. Cord 25 (OH) (nmol/L)

	Treatment			Control				Mean Difference
Study or Subgroup	Mean	SD	Total	Mean	SD	Total	Weight	IV, Random, 95% CI
Corcoy, 2020	75.5	21.9	79	52.8	20.8	75	8.4%	22.70 [15.96, 29.44]
Grant, 2014	62.79	10.93	173	33.12	6.49	63	8.7%	29.67 [27.39, 31.95]
Hashemipour, 2013	69.25	13	55	27.25	11	54	8.6%	42.00 [37.48, 46.52]
Hollis, 2011	24.61	10.19	239	18.2	10.1	111	8.7%	6.41 [4.13, 8.69]
Kalra, 2012	27.34	8.66	96	19.2	5.65	48	8.7%	8.14 [5.78, 10.50]
Mojibian, 2015	94.75	45	186	74.25	47.5	203	8.2%	20.50 [11.31, 29.69]
O'Callaghan, 2018	47.25	15.07	65	32.9	16.3	32	8.4%	14.35 [7.62, 21.08]
Roth, 2018	56.82	20.04	779	11.93	7.37	259	8.8%	44.89 [43.22, 46.56]
Sahoo, 2017	41.73	15.85	36	17.8	13.5	16	8.3%	23.93 [15.53, 32.33]
Yap, 2014	115	47.5	52	72.5	30	47	7.3%	42.50 [27.00, 58.00]
Yesitepe Mutlu, 2014	68.75	36.65	32	47	24.75	19	7.1%	21.75 [4.87, 38.63]
Yu 2009	27	6.72	120	17.5	2.3	59	8.8%	9.50 [8.16, 10.84]
Total (95% CI)			**1912**			**986**	**100.0%**	**23.66 [13.52, 33.79]**

Heterogeneity: Tau² = 304.68; Chi² = 1492.39, df = 11 (P < 0.00001); I² = 99%
Test for overall effect: Z = 4.58 (P < 0.00001)

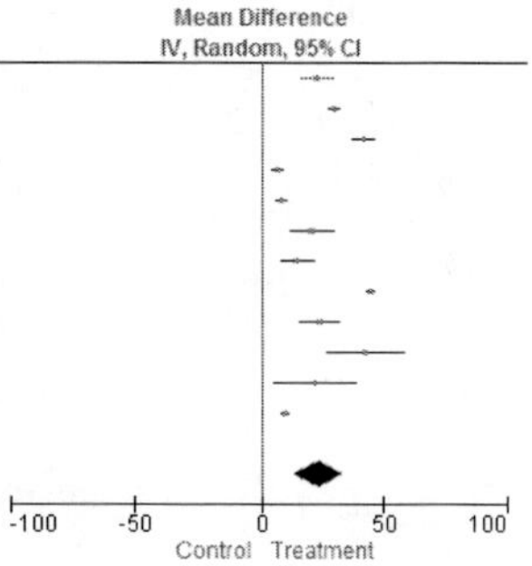

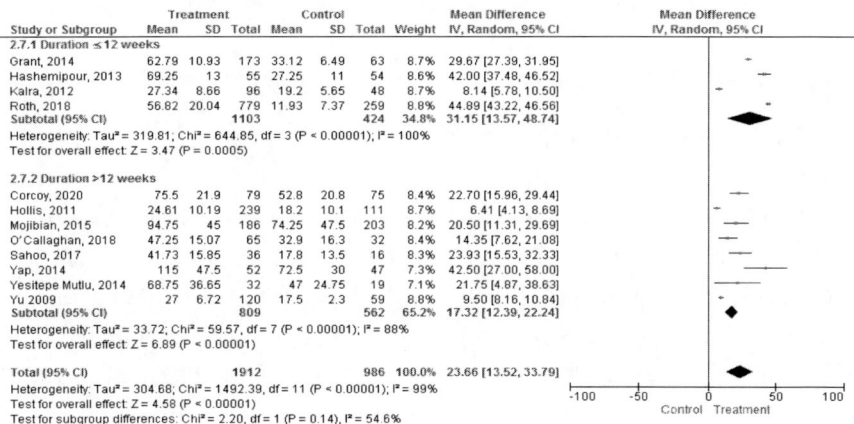

Figure 14. Forest plot on cord 25(OH) D levels (nmol/L).

	Treatment			Control				Mean Difference
Study or Subgroup	Mean	SD	Total	Mean	SD	Total	Weight	IV, Random, 95% CI
2.7.1 Duration ≤ 12 weeks								
Grant, 2014	62.79	10.93	173	33.12	6.49	63	8.7%	29.67 [27.39, 31.95]
Hashemipour, 2013	69.25	13	55	27.25	11	54	8.6%	42.00 [37.48, 46.52]
Kalra, 2012	27.34	8.66	96	19.2	5.65	48	8.7%	8.14 [5.78, 10.50]
Roth, 2018	56.82	20.04	779	11.93	7.37	259	8.8%	44.89 [43.22, 46.56]
Subtotal (95% CI)			1103			424	34.8%	31.15 [13.57, 48.74]
Heterogeneity: Tau² = 319.81; Chi² = 644.85, df = 3 (P < 0.00001); I² = 100%								
Test for overall effect: Z = 3.47 (P = 0.0005)								
2.7.2 Duration >12 weeks								
Corcoy, 2020	75.5	21.9	79	52.8	20.8	75	8.4%	22.70 [15.96, 29.44]
Hollis, 2011	24.61	10.19	239	18.2	10.1	111	8.7%	6.41 [4.13, 8.69]
Mojibian, 2015	94.75	45	186	74.25	47.5	203	8.2%	20.50 [11.31, 29.69]
O'Callaghan, 2018	47.25	15.07	65	32.9	16.3	32	8.4%	14.35 [7.62, 21.08]
Sahoo, 2017	41.73	15.85	36	17.8	13.5	16	8.3%	23.93 [15.53, 32.33]
Yap, 2014	115	47.5	52	72.5	30	47	7.3%	42.50 [27.00, 58.00]
Yesitepe Mutlu, 2014	68.75	36.65	32	47	24.75	19	7.1%	21.75 [4.87, 38.63]
Yu 2009	27	6.72	120	17.5	2.3	59	8.8%	9.50 [8.16, 10.84]
Subtotal (95% CI)			809			562	65.2%	17.32 [12.39, 22.24]
Heterogeneity: Tau² = 33.72; Chi² = 59.57, df = 7 (P < 0.00001); I² = 88%								
Test for overall effect: Z = 6.89 (P < 0.00001)								
Total (95% CI)			**1912**			**986**	**100.0%**	**23.66 [13.52, 33.79]**

Heterogeneity: Tau² = 304.68; Chi² = 1492.39, df = 11 (P < 0.00001); I² = 99%
Test for overall effect: Z = 4.58 (P < 0.00001)
Test for subgroup differences: Chi² = 2.20, df = 1 (P = 0.14), I² = 54.6%

Figure 15. Sub- group analysis of cord 25(OH) D levels based on treatment duration.

The Vitamin D levels in cord blood was found to be adequately high in the neonates born to Vitamin D supplemented mothers. Twelve trials conducted in 2,898 participants were analyzed to obtain a mean difference of 23.66 (95% CI 13.52 to 33.79, I^2 99%). Result of the analysis is presented in Figure 14. Subgroup analysis was conducted based on the treatment duration and sample size. There was not much improvement in the level of heterogeneity; hence no further subgroup analysis was conducted (Figure 15, 16). The results of subgroup analysis are shown in Table 5.

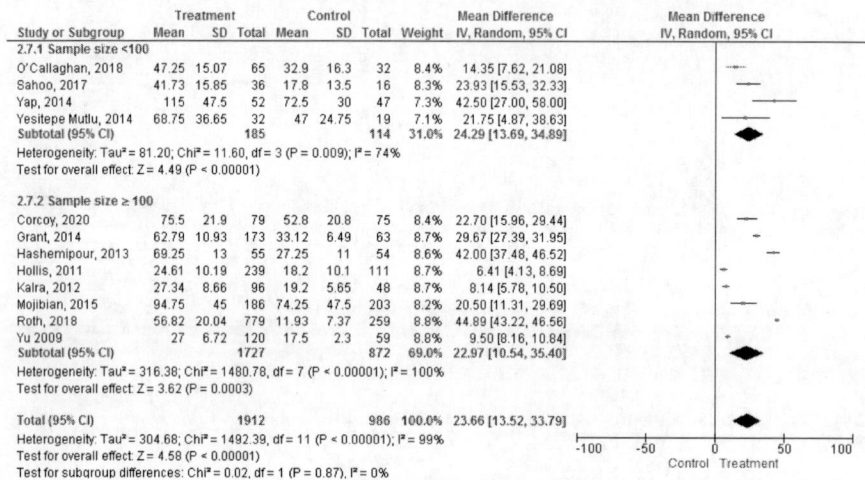

Figure 16. Sub-group analysis of cord 25(OH) D levels based on sample size.

3.2.3.2. Neonatal Anthropometric Measures

Prenatal Vitamin D supplementation did not have any significant effect on neonatal anthropometric measures. The means and standard deviations of birth-weight (g), length (cm) and neonatal head circumference (cm), and were analyzed (Figure 17, 18, 19). In comparison to the control group, the anthropometric measures were high in the Vitamin D supplemented group based on the reports of Hashemipour et al. (2014) [66] and Kalra et al. (2012) [68]. The pooled analysis showed indifference (p = 0.20) in birth-weight between the groups (MD 75.94, 95% CI -41.36 to 193.23, I^2 95%). Data from 9 trials involving 2,226 participants suggested similar head circumference in both the groups (MD 0.20, 95% CI -0.06 to 0.45, I^2 21%). Even neonatal head circumference yielded similar results at p = 0.37 (MD 0.14, 95% CI -0.17 to 0.45, I^2 82%). Subgroup analysis was not conducted for these outcomes due to its insignificant effects.

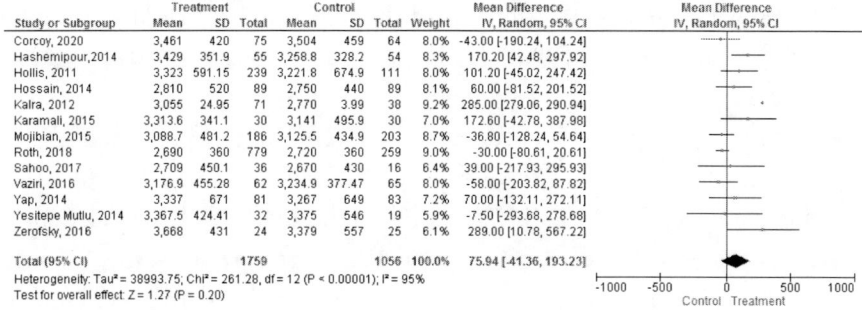

Figure 17. Forest plot on neonatal birth-weight (g).

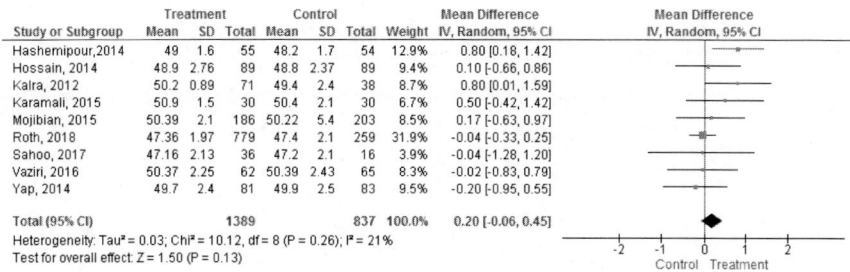

Figure 18. Forest plot on neonatal length (cm).

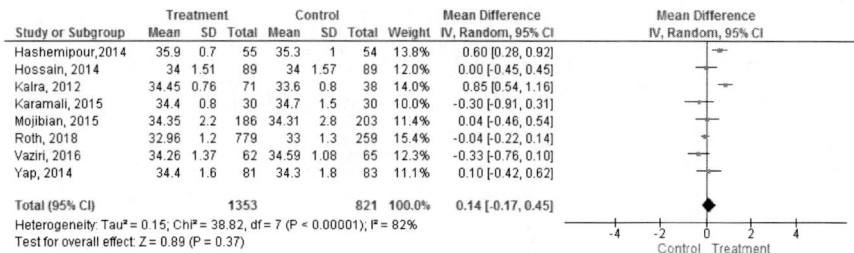

Figure 19. Forest plot on neonatal head circumference (cm).

3.2.4. Safety and Tolerability of Vitamin D Supplementation

Cooper 2016 [82], Corcoy 2020 [83], Dawodu 2013 [64], Enkhmaa 2019 [65], Hollis 2011 [88], Hossain 2014 [67], Rodda 2015 [95], Rostami 2018 [72], Roth 2013 [73], Sablok 2015 [75], Sahu 2009 [77], Shakiba 2013 [78], Wagner 2013 [91] did not find any adverse effects related to Vitamin D supplementation. Mojibian 2015 reported that the serum Vitamin D levels remained within the toxic levels for a dose of 50,000 IU, administered every 2 weeks. In the study by Roth 2018 [74], the distributions of adverse effects were equal in prenatal supplementation and placebo groups. Some participants had experienced mild effects of hypercalcemia and hypercalciuria that did not result in urinary stones or increased hospitalizations. Yap 2014 [96] had also reported mild hypercalcemia in mothers and infants across treatment and control groups (p = 0.13). Nephritic syndrome, nausea and vomiting were reported in two Vitamin D supplemented participants by Yu et al. (2009) [87].

3.3. Effect of Intervention

Table 7. Summary of findings of main outcomes

Outcomes	Anticipated absolute effects* (95% CI)		Relative effect (95% CI)	№ of participants (studies)	Certainty of the evidence (GRADE)
	Risk with placebo or routine low dose vitamin D	Risk with Vitamin D			
Maternal serum 25(OH)D (nmol/L)		MD 31.04 higher (21.33 higher to 40.75 higher)	-	3073 (14 RCTs)	⊕⊕⊕◯ MODERATE [a]
Pre-eclampsia	48 per 1,000	37 per 1,000 (16 to 85)	RR 0.77 (0.34 to 1.76)	1070 (6 RCTs)	⊕⊕◯◯ LOW [b]
GDM	140 per 1,000	102 per 1,000 (71 to 148)	RR 0.73 (0.51 to 1.06)	1096 (5 RCTs)	⊕⊕⊕◯ MODERATE [c]
Cord 25(OH)D (nmol/L)		MD 23.66 higher (13.52 higher to 33.79 higher)	-	2898 (12 RCTs)	⊕⊕◯◯ LOW [d]

Explanations:
a. We downgraded (1) level for serious limitation due to high risk of bias in 3 studies (Kalra 2012, Rodda 2015 and Sahu 2009).
b. We downgraded (2) levels for serious limitation due to high risk of bias in three studies (Ali 2019, Hossain 2014 and Mojibian 2015) and serious limitation in imprecision with wide confidence intervals crossing the clinical decision threshold.
c. We downgraded (1) level for serious limitation due to high risk of bias in three studies (Ali 2019, Hossain 2014 and Mojibian 2015).
d. We downgraded (2) levels for very serious limitations due to high risk of bias in five studies (Hashemipour 2013, Hollis 2011, Kalra 2012, Mojibian 2015 and Yu 200.

The quality of evidence for the main outcomes was determined using GradePro. The four main outcomes had low to moderate quality of evidence. Levels were downgraded due to high risk of bias in some of the included studies. Some studies had reported imprecision due to a wide confidence interval that passed through the threshold of null effect. The summary of findings for changes in the levels of Vitamin D in maternal and cord blood, risk of pre- eclampsia and gestational diabetes is given in Table 7.

4. Discussion

The objective of this chapter is to assess the prevalence of vitamin D deficiency and summarize the published randomized controlled studies on supplementation of vitamin D among pregnant women and report the maternal and neonatal outcomes in the regions of Asia Pacific, United States of America, Europe, Africa, and rest of the world. In this review we have included 34 RCTs and 42 observational studies.

The global prevalence of vitamin D deficiency among pregnant women was estimated and presented based on geographical regions. In the region of Asia 20 observational studies were conducted and the prevalence proportion of vitamin D deficiency among the pregnant women was prominently witnessed with 82.47% In Indonesia, only one study was conducted by Ali et al. 2019 [21] during the dry season, and the pregnant women are likely to have vitamin D deficiency due to limited outdoor activity as a result of morning sickness and women very few women consume the vitamin supplements. And it was found in the study there was a positive correlation between the vitamin D deficiency and the sun exposure. In India, 7 observational studies were conducted, 4 studies (Fareed et al. 2019., Prasad et al. 2018., Sachan et al. 2005 [34]., and Yadav et al, 2018) [25, 32, 34, 38] were conducted in the northern region, one in the western region (Agarwal et al. 2016) [20], one in the eastern region (Sharma et al. 2019) [35] and one in the southern region (Nageshu et al. 2016) [29] of India. The studies conducted in India reported the prevalence of vitamin D deficiency in the population is mostly due to consumption of vegetarian diet, skin pigmentation is dark in color, practicing purdah in the women population expect in the southern region and the vitamin D supplementation is not the part of the routine prescription during the antenatal care of pregnancy. In the regions of the middle east one study is conducted in Saudi Arabia by Aly et al. 2013., [22] and it reported the prevalence of vitamin D deficiency in the pregnant women was due to low socio-economic status, least exposure to sunlight and if the women had two or more pervious births. Two studies in Turkey (Ocal et al. 2019., and Ozdemir et al. 2018) [30, 31] reported the prevalence of vitamin D deficiency and the winter season, low educational status, covered clothing, and the population with low socio-economic status among the pregnant women were the risk factors of prevalence of vitamin D deficiency. One study is conducted in Nepal (Shrestha et al. 2019) [36] mentioned the regular use of supplementation of vitamin D_3 of 250 IU after the first trimester but still there was prevalence of deficiency. There are two study conducted in the region of Thailand (Charatcharoenwitthaya et al. 2013 and Pratumvinit et al. 2015), [23, 33] found the prevalence was high among the pregnant women, who did not consume vitamin fortified milk and did not take prenatal vitamin supplements. One study in South Korea (Choi et al. 2015) [24] and one study in Malaysia and 3 studies conducted in China (Ganmaa et al. 2014., Hong Bi et al. 2018., and Yun et al. 2017) [26-27, 39]. The prevalence is high in pregnant population as most of them limit the sun exposure, use sunscreen to prevent tanning and the Hui ethnicity exhibit high prevalence. In the region of Europe 13 studies were conducted, and proportion of the prevalence was found to be 51.46% and it was significant. The reasons of prevalence of vitamin D deficiency was due to seasons, smoking habits, those who do not consume supplements & vitamin D fortified food products, variations in the UVB exposure at different seasons with respect to the latitude the regions falls.

9 studies were conducted and accounted under the rest of world. Two studies are conducted in Australia (Davies Tuck et al. 2015 and Jones et al. 2016) [53, 55], One in Africa (Figueredo et al. 2018) [54], 4 studies in Canada [56-59] and 2 studies in USA (Hamilton et al. 2010 and Luque Fernandez 2013) [60-61]. The proportion of prevalence was 61.9% with significant deficiency. In the studies conducted in Canada the prevalence

was high because the food chain has limited natural or fortified food resources with vitamin. In USA, due to high latitude and cold climatic conditions the prevalence of deficiency of vitamin is high. In Australia, the vitamin deficiency is due to increase in obesity during pregnancy and seasonal variations. In Africa, the deficiency of vitamin D is attributed to increase on the metabolism of 25(OH)D.

34 published randomized controlled studies were included to assess the supplementation of vitamin D among pregnant women and their maternal and neonatal outcomes in the regions of Asia Pacific, United States of America, Europe, Africa, and rest of the world. 14 Studies were included to assess the levels of vitamin D in the pregnant women who were supplemented with vitamin D_3 irrespective of any dose strength when compared with the population to no intervention or placebo. Maternal 25 (OH) D levels had improved significantly in the vitamin D_3 supplemented group (MD 31.04, 95% CI 21.33 to 40.75). This improvement could be due to different doses and frequency used in the 14 randomized studies and difference in methods of analysis the biomarker. Thus, it is important to interpret the result cautiously.

Further the subgroup analysis was performed to assess the levels of 25(OH)D based on the different doses regimes, Three studies used the dose less than 1000 IU, 6 studies used the dose ranging from 1000 IU to 4000 IU and 5 studies administered the dose greater than 4000 IU. The treatment of duration was assessed for less than 12 weeks and more than 12 weeks period for 14 studies. The sample size based on less than 100 and more than 100 was also evaluated. Thus, it was found that there was improvement in the levels of 25(OH)D in the intervention group among the pregnant women who received the vitamin D_3 supplementation.

The subgroup analysis was performed to assess the vitamin D_3 supplementation effect in the different regions. In Europe, the over effect was 5.51, 1.74 in South Asia, 2.54 in western Asia and 10.64 in other regions. And the overall effect was 6.26. As per most of the guidelines mentions administration of 2000 IU of vitamin D_3 or less among the pregnant women, for which a subgroup to analyze the levels of 25(OH)D in the group less than 2000 IU and more than 2000 IU supplemented with vitamin D_3 and the overall effect size was found to be 7.71 in the group supplemented with more than 2000 IU without any condition of hypervitaminosis and any other adverse effects. The subgroup analysis was performed the evaluate the effect of vitamin D supplementation in prevention of pre-eclampsia and gestational diabetes. The overall effect indicated indifference in the risk of pre-eclampsia (RR 0.77, 95% CI 0.34 to 1.76) and gestational diabetes (RR 0.73, 95% CI 0.51 to 1.06) respectively in treatment and control group. It is mentioned that is when there is vitamin D deficiency there a risk factor involved with endothelial dysfunction and vascular impairment, as vitamin D is a endocrine suppressor on the cells and regulate the renin-angiotensin system there by controlling the blood pressure. Vitamin D modulates the adipokines synthesis which are the factors related to endothelial and vascular health. Thus, there is further need of having enough data to evaluate the effect of vitamin D supplementation in preventing preeclampsia in pregnancy is still inconclusive [97]. Adequate levels of 25(OH)D will increase the sensitivity of the insulin by stimulating the insulin receptor and gene expression and thus increases the insulin mediated glucose transport. Additionally, vitamin D ensure the calcium flux across the cell membranes, which is insulin-mediated intracellular signaling in insulin-responsive tissues. There by 25(OH)D levels plays an important role in the pathogenesis of diabetes mellitus type 2 by affecting insulin sensitivity of β cell function. Thus, it is important to have the highest level of evidence to evaluate the intervention of vitamin D supplementation among the pregnant women to reduce the risk of developing gestational diabetes accounting numerous confounding factors [98]. With respect to the safety outcomes, Vitamin D supplementation during pregnancy did not show any adverse pregnancy outcomes, but if the dose is around 50,000 IU when administered every two weeks the toxic levels were found as reported in the study Mojibian et al. 2015 [70].

With respect to the neonatal outcomes, the analysis was performed on the estimation of cord 25 (OH)D levels, and further subgroup analysis was performed to estimate the cord 25(OH)D levels based on duration and sample size. 25 (OH)D levels in cord blood was found to be adequately high in the neonates born to vitamin D supplemented mothers. Whereas the prenatal Vitamin D supplementation did not have any significant effect on neonatal anthropometric measures. More clinical trials are needed to evaluate the outcomes as not all the outcomes are measure in all studies.

Most of the studies included had missing factor of information of pre gestational BMI and skin pigmentation details which are the determinants of 25(OH)D levels. It is important to have more clinical trials which need to be started early in pregnancy as the effects of supplementation of vitamin before 20 weeks of gestation is more beneficial as it acts on the enzyme the enzyme 1-alpha-hydroxylase, which catalysis the synthesis of 1,25 dihydroxy vitamin D3, has the highest level of expression in the first trimester and it is reduced towards the third trimester.

CONCLUSION

The prevalence proportion of the vitamin D deficiency is found majorly in Asia with 82.4% (95% CI 76.01 to 88.10), the model was statistically significant at $p < 0.001$ and a high heterogeneity of 96.71%. Vitamin D_3 supplementation during pregnancy showed the overall effect in improvement in maternal 25(OH) levels. The overall effect in prevention of pre-eclampsia and gestation diabetes was no different in the vitamin D_3 supplementation group or placebo group. With respect to the neonatal outcomes the 25(OH)D levels in cord blood was found to be high in the neonates born to mothers who were supplemented vitamin D_3 but did not have any significant effect on neonatal anthropometric measures. High quality and rigorous clinical trial studies are required to assess the effects supplementation of vitamin D_3 among the pregnant women and to evaluate the risk associate with it with respect to maternal and neonatal outcomes.

ACKNOWLEDGMENTS

The authors are thankful to JSS College of Pharmacy, Ooty for the assistance and facilitation provided.

REFERENCES

[1] Holick_MF. (2009). Vitamin D status: measurement, interpretation and clinical application. *Annals of Epidemiology:* 19:73-8.

[2] DeLuca, Hector F. (2004)."Overview of General Physiologic Features and Functions of Vitamin D." *The American Journal of Clinical Nutrition* 80 (6) Suppl: 1689–96.

[3] Basutkar, Roopa Satyanarayan, Thomas Eipe, Tenzin Tsundue, Divya Perumal, and Sivasankaran Ponnusankar. (2018). Reduced Vitamin D Levels and Iron Deficiency Anaemia in Pregnant Women: An Evolving Correlation. *Journal of Young Pharmacists* 11 (1): 92–96.

[4] Jones, Glenville. (2008). Pharmacokinetics of Vitamin D Toxicity. *American Journal of Clinical Nutrition* 88 (2): 582–86.

[5] Institute of Medicine (IOM). (2011). *Dietary Reference Intakes for Calcium and Vitamin D.* 2nd Edition. Washington DC: National Academy Press.

[6] Maghbooli, Zhila, Arash Hossein-Nezhad, Ali Reza Shafaei, Farzaneh Karimi, Farzaneh Sadat Madani, and Bagher Larijani. (2007). Vitamin D Status in Mothers and Their Newborns in Iran." *BMC Pregnancy and Childbirth* 7: 1–6.

[7] Clemens, T. L., Henderson S. L, Adams J. S, and Holick M. F. (1997). Increased Skin Pigment Reduces the Capacity of Skin to Synthesis Vitamin D3. *The Lancet*, 74–76.

[8] Ohta, Hiroaki, Tatsuhiko Kuroda, Yoshiko Onoe, Seiya Orito, Mami Ohara, Miyoko Kume, Akiko Harada, Naoko Tsugawa, Toshio Okano, and Satoshi Sasaki. (2009). The Impact of Lifestyle Factors on Serum 25-Hydroxyvitamin D Levels: A Cross-Sectional Study in Japanese Women Aged 19-25 Years. *Journal of Bone and Mineral Metabolism* 27(6): 682–88.

[9] Holick, Michael F., Tai C. Chen, Zhiren Lu, and Edward Sauter. (2007). Vitamin D and Skin Physiology: A D-Lightful Story. *Journal of Bone and Mineral Research* 22 (2): 28–33.

[10] Vimaleswaran, Karani S., Diane J. Berry, Chen Lu, Emmi Tikkanen, Stefan Pilz, Linda T. Hiraki, Jason D. Cooper, et al. (2013). Causal

Relationship between Obesity and Vitamin D Status: Bi-Directional Mendelian Randomization Analysis of Multiple Cohorts. *PLoS Medicine.* 10 (2): e1001383.

[11] Palacios_C, Trak-Fellermeier_MA, Martinez_RX, Lopez-Perez_L, Lips_P, Salisi_JA, John_JC, Peña-Rosas_JP. (2019). Regimens of vitamin D supplementation for women during pregnancy. *Cochrane Database of Systematic Reviews*, Issue 10. Art. No.: CD013446.

[12] Basutkar, Roopa S., Thomas Eipe, Divya Perumal, Prince Wilfred, Kezia K. Sam, Regil C. Varghese, and Sivasankaran Ponnusankar. (2020). Effect of Daily Oral Supplementation of Vitamin D3 in Iron and 25 Hydroxyvitamin d Deficient Pregnant Women: A Randomized Placebo-Controlled Study." *Latin American Journal of Pharmacy* 39 (2): 318–30.

[13] 13. Bodnar, Lisa M., Janet M. Catov, Hyagriv N. Simhan, Michael F. Holick, Robert W. Powers, and James M. Roberts. (2007). Maternal Vitamin D Deficiency Increases the Risk of Preeclampsia. *Journal of Clinical Endocrinology and Metabolism* 92 (9): 3517–22.

[14] Farrant, H. J. W., G. V. Krishnaveni, J. C. Hill, B. J. Boucher, D. J. Fisher, K. Noonan, C. Osmond, S. R. Veena, and C. H. D. Fall. (2009). Vitamin D Insufficiency Is Common in Indian Mothers but Is Not Associated with Gestational Diabetes or Variation in Newborn Size. *European Journal of Clinical Nutrition* 63 (5) (2009): 646–52.

[15] Scholl, Theresa O., Xinhua Chen, and Peter Stein. (2012). Maternal Vitamin D Status and Delivery by Cesarean." *Nutrients* 4 (4): 319–30.

[16] Ford, J. A., D. C. Davidson, W. B. McIntosh, W. M. Fyfe, and M. G. Dunnigan. (1973). Neonatal Rickets in Asian Immigrant Population." *British Medical Journal* 3 (5873): 211–12.

[17] World Health Organization and Food and Agriculture Organization. (2004). *Vitamin and Mineral Requirements in Human Nutrition. 2nd Edition.* Geneva: WHO.

[18] Royal College of Obstetricians and Gynaecologists. (2014). *Vitamin D in Pregnancy. Scientific Impact Paper* https://www.rcog.org.uk/globalassets/documents/guidelines/scientific-impact-papers/vitamin_d_sip43_june14.pdf, Vol. No. 43:1-11.

[19] Hozo, Stela Pudar, Benjamin Djulbegovic, and Iztok Hozo. (2005). Estimating the Mean and Variance from the Median, Range, and the Size of a Sample. *BMC Medical Research Methodology* 5: 1–10.
[20] Agarwal, Shraddha, Minal Chaudhary, Jigisha Chauhan, and Ashwin Vacchani. (2016). Assessment of Vitamin D Deficiency in Pregnant Females Attending Antenatal Care Clinic at Tertiary Care Hospital. *International Journal of Scientific Study* 4 (5): 99–101.
[21] Ali, Aisha Mansoor, Abdulaziz Alobaid, Tasnim Nidal Malhis, and Ahmad Fawzi Khattab. (2019). Effect of Vitamin D3 Supplementation in Pregnancy on Risk of Pre-Eclampsia – Randomized Controlled Trial." *Clinical Nutrition* 38 (2) : 557–63.
[22] Aly, Yasser F, Mohamed A El Koumi, Rehab N Abd, and El Rahman. (2013). *Impact of maternal vitamin D status during pregnancy on the prevalence of neonatal vitamin D deficiency.* 5: e6.
[23] Charatcharoenwitthaya, Natthinee, Tongta Nanthakomon, Charintip Somprasit, Athita Chanthasenanont, La Or Chailurkit, Junya Pattaraarchachai, and Boonsong Ongphiphadhanakul. (2013). Maternal Vitamin D Status, Its Associated Factors and the Course of Pregnancy in Thai Women." *Clinical Endocrinology* 78 (1): 126–33.
[24] Choi, Rihwa, Seonwoo Kim, Heejin Yoo, Yoon Young Cho, Sun Wook Kim, Jae Hoon Chung, Soo Young Oh, and Soo Youn Lee. (2015). High Prevalence of Vitamin D Deficiency in Pregnant Korean Women: The First Trimester and the Winter Season as Risk Factors for Vitamin D Deficiency. *Nutrients* 7 (5): 3427–48.
[25] Fareed, Perveen. (2019). *Assessment of Prevalence Of Vitamin D Deficiency in Pregnant Females in a Tertiary Care Hospital iN Kashmir*" 18 (4): 36–38.
[26] Ganmaa, Davaasambuu, Michael F. Holick, Janet W. Rich-Edwards, Lindsay A. Frazier, Dambadarjaa Davaalkham, Boldbaatar Ninjin, Craig Janes, Robert N. Hoover, and Rebecca Troisi. (2014). Vitamin D Deficiency in Reproductive Age Mongolian Women: A Cross Sectional Study. *Journal of Steroid Biochemistry and Molecular Biology.* 139: 1–6.

[27] Hong-Bi, Song, Xu Yin, Yang Xiaowu, Wang Ying, Xu Yang, Cao Ting, and Wei Na. (2018). High Prevalence of Vitamin D Deficiency in Pregnant Women and Its Relationship with Adverse Pregnancy Outcomes in Guizhou, China. *Journal of International Medical Research* 46 (11) : 4500–4505.
[28] Harleen Kaur. (2019). Prevalence of Vitamin D Deficiency in Pregnant Women. *Journal of Medical Science And Clinical Research* 7 (4): 36–39.
[29] Nageshu, Shailaja, Kirtan Krishna, Krishna L., B. Bhat, H. Suma, and Surekha Reddy. (2016). A Study of Prevalence of Vitamin D Deficiency among Pregnant Women and Its Impact on Feto Maternal Outcome." *International Journal of Reproduction, Contraception, Obstetrics and Gynecology* 5 (4): 1174–80.
[30] Öcal, Doğa F., Zehra Aycan, Gülşah Dağdeviren, Nuray Kanbur, Tuncay Küçüközkan, and Orhan Derman. (2019). Vitamin D Deficiency in Adolescent Pregnancy and Obstetric Outcomes. *Taiwanese Journal of Obstetrics and Gynecology* 58 (6): 778–83.
[31] Özdemir, Abdurrahman Avar, Yasemin Ercan Gündemir, Mustafa Küçük, Deniz Yıldıran Sarıcı, Yusuf Elgörmüş, Yakup Çağ, and Günal Bilek. (2018). Vitamin D Deficiency in Pregnant Women and Their Infants." *JCRPE Journal of Clinical Research in Pediatric Endocrinology* 10 (1): 44–50.
[32] Prasad, Dipali, Kalpana Singh, and Swet Nisha. (2018). *Section : Obstetrics and Gynecology Vitamin D in Pregnancy and Its Correlation with Feto Maternal Outcome Section: Obstetrics and Gynecology* 5 (1): 1–5.
[33] Pratumvinit, Busadee, Preechaya Wongkrajang, Tuangsit Wataganara, Sithikan Hanyongyuth, Akarin Nimmannit, Somruedee Chatsiricharoenkul, Kotchamol Manonukul, and Kanit Reesukumal.(2015). Maternal Vitamin d Status and Its Related Factors in Pregnant Women in Bangkok, Thailand. *PLoS ONE*. 10 (7): 1–14.
[34] Alok Sachan, Renu Gupta, Vinita Das, Anjoo Agarwal, Pradeep K Awasthi, and Vijayalakshmi Bhatia. (2005). High prevalence of

vitamin D deficiency among pregnant women and their newborns in northern India. *Am J Clin Nutr* 81: 1060.

[35] Sharma N, Nath C, Mohammad J. (2019). Vitamin D status in pregnant women visiting a tertiary care center of North Eastern India. *J Family Med Prim Care*, 8:356-60.

[36] Dhruba Shrestha, Saraswati Budhathoki, Sabi Pokhrel, Ashok Kumar Sah, Raj Kumar Shrestha, Ganendra Bhakta Raya et al., (2019). Prevalence of vitamin D deficiency in pregnant women and their babies in Bhaktapur, Nepal. *BMC Nutrition*:5:31.

[37] Woon, Fui Chee, Yit Siew Chin, Intan Hakimah Ismail, Marijka Batterham, Amir Hamzah Abdul Latiff, Wan Ying Gan, Geeta Appannah, et al. (2019). Vitamin D Deficiency during Pregnancy and Its Associated Factors among Third Trimester Malaysian Pregnant Women. *PLoS ONE* 14 (6): 1–12.

[38] Yadav, Munmun, Mahendra Kumar Verma, Mohan Bairwa, Govardhan Meena, and Lata Rajoria.(2018). Prevalence of Vitamin D Deficiency and Effect of Vitamin D Supplementation on Feto-Maternal Outcome in Tertiary Care Centre. *International Journal of Reproduction, Contraception, Obstetrics and Gynecology* 7 (12): 4912.

[39] Yun, Chunfeng, Jing Chen, Yuna He, Deqian Mao, Rui Wang, Yu Zhang, Chun Yang, Jianhua Piao, and Xiaoguang Yang. (2017). Vitamin D Deficiency Prevalence and Risk Factors among Pregnant Chinese Women. *Public Health Nutrition* 20 (10): 1746–54.

[40] Brembeck, Petra, Anna Winkvist, and Hanna Olausson. (2013). Determinants of Vitamin D Status in Pregnant Fair-Skinned Women in Sweden. *British Journal of Nutrition* 110 (5): 856–64.

[41] Cabaset, Sophie, Jean-Philippe Krieger, Aline Richard, Magdeldin Elgizouli, Alexandra Nieters, Sabine Rohrmann, and Katharina C. Quack Lötscher. (2019). Vitamin D Status and Its Determinants in Healthy Pregnant Women Living in Switzerland in the First Trimester of Pregnancy. *BMC Pregnancy and Childbirth* 19 (1): 1–12.

[42] Dovnik, Andraž, Faris Mujezinović, Milena Treiber, Breda Pečovnik Balon, Maksimiljan Gorenjak, Uroš Maver, and Iztok Takač. (2014).

Seasonal Variations of Vitamin D Concentrations in Pregnant Women and Neonates in Slovenia. *European Journal of Obstetrics and Gynecology and Reproductive Biology* 181: 6–9.

[43] Emmerson, Anthoney J. B., Karen Elizabeth Dockery, M. Z. Mughal, Stephen A. Roberts, Clare Louise Tower, and Jacqueline L. Berry. (2018). Vitamin D Status of White Pregnant Women and Infants at Birth and 4 Months in North West England: A Cohort Study. *Maternal and Child Nutrition* 14 (1): 1–11.

[44] Haggarty, Paul, Doris M. Campbell, Susan Knox, Graham W. Horgan, Gwen Hoad, Emma Boulton, Geraldine McNeill, and Alan M. Wallace. (2013). Vitamin D in Pregnancy at High Latitude in Scotland. *British Journal of Nutrition* 109 (5): 898–905.

[45] Holmes, Valerie A., Maria S. Barnes, H. Denis Alexander, Peter McFaul, and Julie M. W. Wallace. (2009). Vitamin D Deficiency and Insufficiency in Pregnant Women: A Longitudinal Study. *British Journal of Nutrition* 102 (6): 876–81.

[46] Skowrońska-Jóźwiak, Elzbieta, Zbigniew Adamczewski, Agnieszka Tyszkiewicz, Kinga Krawczyk-Rusiecka, Krzysztof Lewandowski, and Andrzej Lewiński. (2014). Assessment of Adequacy of Vitamin D Supplementation during Pregnancy. *Annals of Agricultural and Environmental Medicine.* 21(1): 198-200.

[47] Krieger, Jean Philippe, Sophie Cabaset, Claudia Canonica, Ladina Christoffel, Aline Richard, Therese Schröder, Begoña Lipp Von Wattenwyl, Sabine Rohrmann, and Katharina Quack Lötscher. (2018). Prevalence and Determinants of Vitamin D Deficiency in the Third Trimester of Pregnancy: A Multicentre Study in Switzerland. *British Journal of Nutrition* 119 (3): 299–309.

[48] Lundqvist, Anette, Herbert Sandström, Hans Stenlund, Ingegerd Johansson, and Johan Hultdin. (2016). Vitamin D Status during Pregnancy: A Longitudinal Study in Swedish Women from Early Pregnancy to Seven Months Postpartum. *PLoS ONE* 11 (3): 1–12.

[49] Mcaree, Trixie, Benjamin Jacobs, Thubeena Manickavasagar, Suganthinie Sivalokanathan, Lauren Brennan, Paul Bassett, Sandra Rainbow, and Mitch Blair. (2013). Vitamin D Deficiency in Pregnancy

- Still a Public Health Issue." *Maternal and Child Nutrition* 9 (1): 23–30.
[50] Nicolaidou, P., Z. Hatzistamatiou, A. Papadopoulou, J. Kaleyias, E. Floropoulou, E. Lagona, V. Tsagris, C. Costalos, and A. Antsaklis. (2006). Low Vitamin D Status in Mother-Newborn Pairs in Greece." *Calcified Tissue International* 78 (6): 337–42.
[51] Rodriguez, Agueda, Loreto Santa Marina, Ana María Jimenez, Ana Esplugues, Ferran Ballester, Mercedes Espada, Jordi Sunyer, and Eva Morales. (2016). Vitamin D Status in Pregnancy and Determinants in a Southern European Cohort Study. *Paediatric and Perinatal Epidemiology* 30 (3): 217–28.
[52] Vandevijvere, Stefanie, Sihame Amsalkhir, Herman van Oyen, and Rodrigo Moreno-Reyes. (2012). High Prevalence of Vitamin D Deficiency in Pregnant Women: A National Cross-Sectional Survey. *PLoS ONE* 7 (8): 1–9.
[53] Davies-Tuck, Miranda, Cheryl Yim, Michelle Knight, Ryan Hodges, James C. G. Doery, and Euan Wallace. (2015). Vitamin D Testing in Pregnancy: Does One Size Fit All?. *Australian and New Zealand Journal of Obstetrics and Gynaecology* 55 (2): 149–55.
[54] Figueiredo, Amanda C. Cunha, Paula Guedes Cocate, Amanda R. Amorim Adegboye, Ana Beatriz Franco-Sena, Dayana R. Farias, Maria Beatriz Trindade de Castro, Alex Brito, et al. (2018). Changes in Plasma Concentrations of 25-Hydroxyvitamin D and 1,25-Dihydroxyvitamin D during Pregnancy: A Brazilian Cohort. *European Journal of Nutrition* 57 (3): 1059–72.
[55] Jones, A. P., K. Rueter, A. Siafarikas, E. M. Lim, S. L. Prescott, and D. J. Palmer. (2016). 25-Hydroxyvitamin D Status of Pregnant Women Is Associated with the Use of Antenatal Vitamin Supplements and Ambient Ultraviolet Radiation. *Journal of Developmental Origins of Health and Disease* 7 (4): 350–56.
[56] Kramer, Caroline K., Chang Ye, Balakumar Swaminathan, Anthony J. Hanley, Philip W. Connelly, Mathew Sermer, Bernard Zinman, and Ravi Retnakaran. (2016). The Persistence of Maternal Vitamin D Deficiency and Insufficiency during Pregnancy and Lactation

Irrespective of Season and Supplementation. *Clinical Endocrinology* 84 (5): 680–86.

[57] Perreault, Maude, Caroline J. Moore, Gerhard Fusch, Koon K. Teo, and Stephanie A. Atkinson. (2019). Factors Associated with Serum 25-Hydroxyvitamin d Concentration in Two Cohorts of Pregnant Women in Southern Ontario, Canada. *Nutrients* 11 (1):123.

[58] Shand, A. W., N. Nassar, P. Von Dadelszen, S. M. Innis, and T. J. Green. (2010). Maternal Vitamin D Status in Pregnancy and Adverse Pregnancy Outcomes in a Group at High Risk for Pre-Eclampsia." *BJOG: An International Journal of Obstetrics and Gynaecology* 117 (13): 1593–98.

[59] Wei, S. Q., F. Audibert, N. Hidiroglou, K. Sarafin, P. Julien, Y. Wu, Z. C. Luo, and W. D. Fraser. (2012). Longitudinal Vitamin D Status in Pregnancy and the Risk of Pre-Eclampsia. *BJOG: An International Journal of Obstetrics and Gynaecology* 119 (7): 832–39.

[60] Wagner, Carol L., Stuart A. Hamilton, Rebecca McNeil, Bruce W. Hollis, Deborah J. Davis, Joyce Winkler, Carolina Cook, Gloria Warner, Betty Bivens, and Patrick McShane. (2010). Profound Vitamin D Deficiency in a Diverse Group of Women during Pregnancy Living in a Sun-Rich Environment at Latitude 32N. *International Journal of Endocrinology.* 917428.

[61] Luque-Fernandez, Miguel Angel, Bizu Gelaye, Tyler Vanderweele, Cynthia Ferre, Anna Maria Siega-Riz, Claudia Holzman, Daniel A. Enquobahrie, Nancy Dole, and Michelle A. Williams. (2014). Seasonal Variation of 25-Hydroxyvitamin D among Non-Hispanic Black and White Pregnant Women from Three US Pregnancy Cohorts. *Paediatric and Perinatal Epidemiology* 28 (2): 166–76.

[62] Ali, Aisha Mansoor, Abdulaziz Alobaid, Tasnim Nidal Malhis, and Ahmad Fawzi Khattab. (2019). Effect of Vitamin D3 Supplementation in Pregnancy on Risk of Pre-Eclampsia – Randomized Controlled Trial." *Clinical Nutrition* 38 (2) : 557–63.

[63] Asemi, Zatollah, Mansooreh Samimi, Zohreh Tabassi, Hossein Shakeri, and Ahmad Esmaillzadeh. (2013). Vitamin D Supplementation Affects Serum High-Sensitivity C-Reactive Protein,

Insulin Resistance, and Biomarkers of Oxidative Stress in Pregnant Women. *Journal of Nutrition* 143 (9): 1432–38.

[64] Dawodu, Adekunle, Hussein F. Saadi, Gharid Bekdache, Yasin Javed, Mekibib Altaye, and Bruce W. Hollis.(2013). Randomized Controlled Trial (RCT) of Vitamin D Supplementation in Pregnancy in a Population with Endemic Vitamin D Deficiency. *Journal of Clinical Endocrinology and Metabolism* 98 (6): 2337–46.

[65] Enkhmaa, D., L. Tanz, D. Ganmaa, Sh Enkhtur, B. Oyun-Erdene, J. Stuart, G. Chen, et al. (2019). Randomized Trial of Three Doses of Vitamin D to Reduce Deficiency in Pregnant Mongolian Women. *EBioMedicine* 39 (xxxx): 510–19.

[66] Hashemipour, Sima, Amir Ziaee, Amir Javadi, Farideh Movahed, Khadijeh Elmizadeh, Ezzatalsadat Hajiseid Javadi, and Fatemeh Lalooha. (2014). Effect of Treatment of Vitamin D Deficiency and Insufficiency during Pregnancy on Fetal Growth Indices and Maternal Weight Gain: A Randomized Clinical Trial." *European Journal of Obstetrics and Gynecology and Reproductive Biology* 172 (1) (2014): 15–19.

[67] Hossain, Nazli, Fatima H. Kanani, Shabana Ramzan, Robina Kausar, Shabana Ayaz, Rafiq Khanani, and Lubna Pal.(2014). Obstetric and Neonatal Outcomes of Maternal Vitamin D Supplementation: Results of an Open-Label, Randomized Controlled Trial of Antenatal Vitamin D Supplementation in Pakistani Women. *Journal of Clinical Endocrinology and Metabolism* 99 (7): 2448–55.

[68] Kalra, Pramila, Vinita Das, Anjoo Agarwal, Mala Kumar, V. Ramesh, Eesh Bhatia, Sarika Gupta, Swati Singh, Priya Saxena, and Vijayalakshmi Bhatia. (2012). Effect of Vitamin D Supplementation during Pregnancy on Neonatal Mineral Homeostasis and Anthropometry of the Newborn and Infant. *British Journal of Nutrition* 108 (6): 1052–58.

[69] Karamali, M., E. Beihaghi, A. A. Mohammadi, and Z. Asemi. (2015). "Effects of High-Dose Vitamin D Supplementation on Metabolic Status and Pregnancy Outcomes in Pregnant Women at Risk for Pre-

Eclampsia. (2015). *Hormone and Metabolic Research* 47 (12): 867–72.

[70] Mojibian, Mahdieh, Sedigheh Soheilykhah, Mohammad Ali Fallah Zadeh, and Maryam Jannati Moghadam. (2015). The Effects of Vitamin D Supplementation on Maternal and Neonatal Outcome: A Randomized Clinical Trial." *International Journal of Reproductive BioMedicine* 13 (11) : 687–96.

[71] Motamed, Soudabe, Bahareh Nikooyeh, Maryam Kashanian, Bruce W. Hollis, and Tirang R. Neyestani. (2019). Efficacy of Two Different Doses of Oral Vitamin D Supplementation on Inflammatory Biomarkers and Maternal and Neonatal Outcomes." *Maternal and Child Nutrition* 15 (4): 1–10.

[72] Rostami, Maryam, Fahimeh Ramezani Tehrani, Masoumeh Simbar, Razieh Bidhendi Yarandi, Sonia Minooee, Bruce W. Hollis, and Farhad Hosseinpanah. (2018). Effectiveness of Prenatal Vitamin D Deficiency Screening and Treatment Program: A Stratified Randomized Field Trial." *Journal of Clinical Endocrinology and Metabolism* 103 (8): 2936–48.

[73] Roth, Daniel E., Abdullah Al Mahmud, Rubhana Raqib, Evana Akhtar, Nandita Perumal, Brendon Pezzack, and Abdullah H. Baqui. (2013). Randomized Placebo-Controlled Trial of High-Dose Prenatal Third-Trimester Vitamin D3 Supplementation in Bangladesh: The AViDD Trial." *Nutrition Journal* 12(1): 1–16.

[74] Roth, D. E., S. K. Morris, S. Zlotkin, A. D. Gernand, T. Ahmed, S. S. Shanta, E. Papp, et al. (2018). Vitamin D Supplementation in Pregnancy and Lactation and Infant Growth. *New England Journal of Medicine* 379 (6): 535–46.

[75] Sablok, Aanchal, Aruna Batra, Karishma Thariani, Achla Batra, Rekha Bharti, Abha Rani AggarwalB. C. Kabi, and Harish Chellani. (2015). Supplementation of Vitamin D in Pregnancy and Its Correlation with Feto-Maternal Outcome." *Clinical Endocrinology* 83 (4): 536–41.

[76] Sahoo, Saroj Kumar, Kishore Kumar Katam, Vinita Das, Anjoo Agarwal, and Vijayalakshmi Bhatia. (2017). Maternal Vitamin D Supplementation in Pregnancy and Offspring Outcomes: A Double-

Blind Randomized Placebo-Controlled Trial. *Journal of Bone and Mineral Metabolism* 35 (4): 464–71.

[77] Sahu, M., V. Das, A. Aggarwal, V. Rawat, P. Saxena, and V. Bhatia. (2009). Vitamin D Replacement in Pregnant Women in Rural North India: A Pilot Study. *European Journal of Clinical Nutrition* 63 (9): 1157–59.

[78] Shakiba, Mehrdad, and Mohamad Reza Iranmanesh. (2013). Vitamin D Requirement in Pregnancy to Prevent Deficiency in Neonates: A Randomised Trial. *Singapore Medical Journal* 54 (5): 285–88.

[79] Vafaei, Homeira, Nasrin Asadi, Maryam Kasraeian, Hadi Raeisi Shahraki, Khadije Bazrafshan, and Niloofar Namazi.(2019). Positive Effect of Low Dose Vitamin D Supplementation on Growth of Fetal Bones: A Randomized Prospective Study. *Bone* 122 (2): 136–42.

[80] Vaziri, Farideh, Mohammad Hossein Dabbaghmanesh, Alamtaj Samsami, Samira Nasiri, and Pedram Talezadeh Shirazi.(2016). Vitamin D Supplementation during Pregnancy on Infant Anthropometric Measurements and Bone Mass of Mother-Infant Pairs: A Randomized Placebo Clinical Trial. *Early Human Development* 103: 61–68.

[81] Mutlu, Gul Yesiltepe, Elif Ozsu, Sibel Kalaca, Aysegul Yuksel, Yuksel Pehlevan, Filiz Cizmecioglu, and Sukru Hatun. (2014). Evaluation of Vitamin D Supplementation Doses during Pregnancy in a Population at High Risk for Deficiency. *Hormone Research in Paediatrics* 81 (6): 402–8.

[82] Cooper, Cyrus, Nicholas C. Harvey, Nicholas J. Bishop, Stephen Kennedy, Aris T. Papageorghiou, Inez Schoenmakers, Robert Fraser, et al. (2016). Maternal Gestational Vitamin D Supplementation and Offspring Bone Health (MAVIDOS): A Multicentre, Double-Blind, Randomised Placebo-Controlled Trial." *The Lancet Diabetes and Endocrinology* 4 (5): 393–402.

[83] Corcoy, Rosa, Lilian C. Mendoza, David Simmons, Gernot Desoye, J. M. Adelantado, Ana Chico, Roland Devlieger, et al. (2020). The DALI Vitamin D Randomized Controlled Trial for Gestational Diabetes

Mellitus Prevention: No Major Benefit Shown besides Vitamin D Sufficiency. *Clinical Nutrition* 39 (3): 976–84.

[84] Moon, Rebecca J, Nicholas C Harvey, Cyrus Cooper, Stefania D Angelo, Sarah R Crozier, Hazel M Inskip, Inez Schoenmakers, et al. (2016). *Determinants of the Maternal 25-Hydroxyvitamin D Response to Vitamin D Supplementation During Pregnancy.* 101 (10): 1–9.

[85] O'callaghan, Karen M., Áine Hennessy, George L. J. Hull, Karina Healy, Christian Ritz, Louise C. Kenny, Kevin D. Cashman, and Mairead E. Kiely. (2018). Estimation of the Maternal Vitamin D Intake That Maintains Circulating 25-HydroxyVitamin D in Late Gestation at a Concentration Sufficient to Keep Umbilical Cord Sera ≥25-30 Nmol/L: A Dose-Response, Double-Blind, Randomized Placebo-Controlled Trial in Pre." *American Journal of Clinical Nutrition* 108 (1): 77–91.

[86] Stoutjesdijk, E, A Schaafsma, I P Kema, J V A N D E R Molen, Friesland Campina, Herman J A Velvis, and Wietske Hemminga. *Influence of daily 10-85 microgram vitamin D supplements during Pregnancy and lactation on maternal vitamin D status and mature Milk anti rachitic activity.* (2018) "Accepted Manuscript."

[87] Yu, C. K. H., L. Sykes, M. Sethi, T. G. Teoh, and S. Robinson. (2009). Vitamin D Deficiency and Supplementation during Pregnancy." *Clinical Endocrinology* 70 (5): 685–90.

[88] Hollis BW, Johnson D, Hulsey TC, Ebeling M, Wagner CL. (2011). Vitamin D supplementation during pregnancy: double-blind, randomized clinical trial of safety and effectiveness. *J Bone Miner Res.*;26(10):2341-2357.

[89] March, Kaitlin M., Nancy N. Chen, Crystal D. Karakochuk, Antonia W. Shand, Sheila M. Innis, Peter Von Dadelszen, Susan I. Barr, et al. (2015). Maternal Vitamin D3 Supplementation at 50 Mg/d Protects against Low Serum 25-Hydroxyvitamin D in Infants at 8 Wk of Age: A Randomized Controlled Trial of 3 Doses of Vitamin D Beginning in Gestation and Continued in Lactation. *American Journal of Clinical Nutrition* 102 (2): 402–10.

[90] Thiele, Doria K., Jody Ralph, Maher El-Masri, and Cindy M. Anderson. (2017). Vitamin D3 Supplementation During Pregnancy and Lactation Improves Vitamin D Status of the Mother–Infant Dyad. *JOGNN - Journal of Obstetric, Gynecologic, and Neonatal Nursing* 46 (1): 135–47.

[91] Wagner, Carol L., Rebecca McNeil, Stuart A. Hamilton, Joyce Winkler, Carolina Rodriguez Cook, Gloria Warner, Betty Bivens, et al. (2013). A Randomized Trial of Vitamin D Supplementation in 2 Community Health Center Networks in South Carolina. *American Journal of Obstetrics and Gynecology* 208 (2): 137.e1-137.e13.

[92] Wei, Wei, Judith R. Shary, Elizabeth Garrett-Mayer, Betsy Anderson, Nina E. Forestieri, Bruce W. Hollis, and Carol L. Wagner. (2017). Bone Mineral Density during Pregnancy in Women Participating in a Randomized Controlled Trial of Vitamin D Supplementation. *American Journal of Clinical Nutrition* 106 (6): 1422–30.

[93] Zerofsky, Melissa S., Bryon N. Jacoby, Theresa L. Pedersen, and Charles B. Stephensen. (2016). Daily Cholecalciferol Supplementation during Pregnancy Alters Markers of Regulatory Immunity, Inflammation, and Clinical Outcomes in a Randomized Controlled Trial." *Journal of Nutrition* 146 (11): 2388–97.

[94] Grant, Cameron C., Alistair W. Stewart, Robert Scragg, Tania Milne, Judy Rowden, Alec Ekeroma, Clare Wall, et al. (2014). Vitamin D during Pregnancy and Infancy and Infant Serum 25-Hydroxyvitamin D Concentration." *Pediatrics* 133(1): e143-153.

[95] Rodda, C. P., J. E. Benson, A. J. Vincent, C. L. Whitehead, A. Polykov, and B. Vollenhoven. (2015). Maternal Vitamin D Supplementation during Pregnancy Prevents Vitamin D Deficiency in the Newborn: An Open-Label Randomized Controlled Trial. *Clinical Endocrinology* 83 (3): 363–68.

[96] Yap, Constance, N. Wah Cheung, Jenny E. Gunton, Neil Athayde, Craig F. Munns, Anna Duke, and Mark McLean. (2014). Vitamin D Supplementation and the Effects on Glucose Metabolism during Pregnancy: A Randomized Controlled Trial. *Diabetes Care* 37 (7): 1837–44.

[97] Fogacci, Silvia, Federica Fogacci, Maciej Banach, Erin D Michos, Adrian V Hernandez, Gregory Y H Lip, Michael J Blaha, et al. (2020). Vitamin D Supplementation and Incident Preeclampsia : A Systematic Review and Meta-Analysis of Randomized Clinical Trials. *Clinical Nutrition* 39 (6): 1742–52.

[98] Anna Pleska, Vendula Bartáková, Lukáš Pácal, Katarína Kuricová, B Jana, and Josef Tomandl. (2015). *Vitamin D Status in Women with Gestational Diabetes Mellitus during Pregnancy and Postpartum.*

In: Vitamin Deficiency ISBN: 978-1-53618-979-7
Editors: N. Stewart and D. Thomson © 2021 Nova Science Publishers, Inc.

Chapter 2

STUDY OF THE ROLE OF VITAMINS K AND D ON THE PROGRESSION OF HUMAN OSTEOSARCOMA BASED ON *IN VITRO* RESULTS

Evangelia Pantazaka[1], PhD,
Angelos Kaspiris[2,*], MD, PhD,
Dimitra Melissaridou[3], MD,
Olga D. Savvidou[3], MD, PhD and
Panayiotis J. Papagelopoulos[3], MD, DSc, FACS

[1]Section of Organic Chemistry and Biochemistry,
Department of Chemistry, University of Patras, Patras, Greece
[2]Laboratory of Molecular Pharmacology,
Section of Orthopaedic Research, School of Health Sciences,
University of Patras, Patras, Greece
[3]First Department of Orthopaedic Surgery,
ATTIKON University Hospital and Medical School,
National and Kapodistrian University of Athens, Athens, Greece

---

* Corresponding Author's E-mail: angkaspiris@hotmail.com.

ABSTRACT

Osteosarcoma is one of the most prevailing, aggressive primary bone tumors, affecting mainly children and younger populations worldwide. The 60-70% patients' survival rate is not deemed satisfactory, and the high metastasis and relapse frequency, further supports the need for more intense efforts towards the identification of novel therapeutics. Vitamin K, a family of vitamins which exist as both natural and synthetic forms, are essential in bone formation and metabolism and act as cofactor for the post-translational γ-carboxylation of bone matrix proteins. Vitamin K studied in osteosarcoma cells have been reported to be transcriptional regulators of bone-specific genes favoring the expression of bone-related markers, to inhibit cell growth and migration, to induce apoptosis of osteosarcoma cells and affect the transition of cell death mode from apoptosis to necrosis. Vitamin D is another family of fat-soluble vitamins. Vitamin D is known for promoting calcium deposition in bones. Both vitamins K and D have also been demonstrated to exert antitumor effects on a plethora of cancer cell lines, yet their role in osteosarcoma is not fully elucidated. This chapter will introduce these essential vitamins, briefly discuss their functions, present the links between them, provide insight on the underlying mechanisms responsible for their role in osteosarcoma and identify future perspectives.

Keywords: osteosarcoma progression, Vitamin K, Vitamin D

INTRODUCTION

It is documented that a vast number of cancer patients take dietary supplements on top of their conventional treatment, so as to avoid and/or postpone a potential relapse. In fact, it appears that >60% of cancer patients and survivors use vitamin and mineral supplements (Davis-Yadley and Malafa 2015). Interestingly, there are currently no established recommendations on the use of vitamins to ameliorate conventional treatment and to prevent recurrence, and/or metastasis in osteosarcoma. In this chapter, literature regarding vitamins, with a focus on vitamins K and D, and their role in osteosarcoma cancer, is explored. These two vitamins were considered to be the most relevant, based on the amount of evidence available and the authors' research interests. Focus was mainly on the relevant *in vitro* studies conducted and the potential role and mechanism of action of these vitamins in osteosarcoma was discussed. Potential future research strategies for osteosarcoma cancer intervention with the use of these vitamins will be proposed.

VITAMIN K

Vitamin K: General Concepts

Vitamin K was discovered approximately 90 years ago. The "discovery of vitamin K" itself and that of its "chemical nature" was awarded the Nobel Prize in Physiology or Medicine in 1943. "K" comes from the word "koagulation" and describes the first and mostly known function of vitamin K, blood coagulation.

Vitamin K is a family of structurally related compounds which share a hydrophilic 2-methyl-1,4-naphthoquinone ring structure and a lipophilic side chain, varying in length and degree of saturation, at the 3-position. The three main types of vitamin K are vitamin K1 (or phylloquinone), vitamin K2 (or menaquinones) and vitamin K3 (or menadione) (Rodriguez-Olleros Rodriguez and Diaz Curiel 2019; Shioi et al. 2020; Simes et al. 2020).

Vitamin K1 is characterized by a phytyl side chain (analogous to that of chlorophyll with four isoprenoid residues of which three are saturated), vitamin K2 consists of a side chain of repeating isoprenoid units (and are hence classified as menaquinone-n, where n is the number of the repeating units and are collectively referred to as vitamin K2), while vitamin K3 lacks a big side chain and only has a methyl group (Rodriguez-Olleros Rodriguez and Diaz Curiel 2019; Palmer et al. 2020; Shioi et al. 2020; Simes et al. 2020; Akbari and Rasouli-Ghahroudi 2018).

Vitamins K1 and K2 are the naturally occurring forms (Rodriguez-Olleros Rodriguez and Diaz Curiel 2019; Palmer et al. 2020; Shioi et al. 2020; Simes et al. 2020, 2019; Akbari and Rasouli-Ghahroudi 2018).

Vitamin K1 is synthesized by plants, algae and cyanobacteria. Vitamin K2 is primarily produced by bacteria present in the human intestine, with the exception of menaquinone-4, the prevalent form of vitamin K in the human body, which is considered to be of animal origin as it is produced in specific tissues following conversion of some of the ingested vitamin K1 into vitamin K3, and its subsequent conversion to menaquinone-4 in the liver. These gut bacteria are responsible for lengthening the molecule's isoprenoid side chain. The longer chain menaquinone-7 can also be converted to the shorter vitamin K2 form, menaquinone-4 (Akbari and Rasouli-Ghahroudi 2018; Azuma and Inoue 2019; Ciebiera et al. 2020). Vitamin K3 is a chemically synthesized, water-soluble form of vitamin K, which can also be converted by the liver into menaquinone-4 (Rodriguez-Olleros Rodriguez and Diaz Curiel 2019; Palmer et al. 2020; Shioi et al. 2020; Simes et al. 2020, 2019; Akbari and Rasouli-Ghahroudi 2018). Vitamin K3 synthetic analogues, such as menadione-4 (2-methyl-1,4-naphthalenediyldiacetate) (Jiang et al. 2013), has been clinically used as hemostasis treatment and its anticancer activity will be discussed below.

Vitamin K is found in food, but can also be a supplement (mostly vitamin K2 and specifically menaquinone-4 and menaquinone-7). Vitamin K1 is the major dietary source of vitamin K, and is abundant in green leafy vegetables, fruit, grains and dairy products (Rodriguez-Olleros Rodriguez and Diaz Curiel 2019). Vitamin K2 is contained in animal-based and fermented food. Vitamin K3 is supplemented in animal food, so as to prevent fractures, and is found in the form of vitamin K2 in the meat of farmed animals (Rodriguez-Olleros Rodriguez and Diaz Curiel 2019; Azuma and Inoue 2019).

Vitamin K: Functions

Vitamins K1 and K2 (but not K3) have been shown to be fundamental as cofactors during the post-translational modification of Glu residues to γ-carboxyglutamic acid (Gla), which bind calcium, for the synthesis of Gla-containing proteins, such as coagulation factors II, VII, IX, X in the liver (by vitamin K1 being transported there), and bone Gla-protein (or osteocalcin, the most abundant bone protein), and matrix Gla-protein at extra-hepatic sites (by vitamin K2 being transported to bone and vascular wall) (Sato et al. 2012; Carr et al. 2002; Ciebiera et al. 2020; Kaneki et al. 2006; Azuma and Inoue 2019; Ivanova et al. 2018; Fusaro et al. 2011; Shioi et al. 2020; Marchili et al. 2018). Deficiency of vitamin K results in the synthesis of under-carboxylated proteins, associated with unfavorable outcomes (Lanham-New 2008).

Vitamin K has been reported to exert a plethora of functions beyond coagulation and the mechanisms involved are gradually being elucidated. Vitamin K supplementation may be useful for numerous conditions afflicting the ageing population, and this could have major impact on relieving the financial burden which accompanies these diseases. Vitamin K is essential for maintaining bone health and metabolism (Tsugawa and Shiraki 2020; Walther et al. 2013; Akbari and Rasouli-Ghahroudi 2018), while vitamin K deficiency has been linked to bone issues such as increased bone fracture risks (Tsugawa and Shiraki 2020; Halder et al. 2019). Clinical evidence suggests that vitamin K could play a protective role on the inflammatory and mineralization processes which are both associated with age-related diseases such as cardiovascular diseases [reviewed in (Simes et al. 2019; Schwalfenberg 2017; Shioi et al. 2020; Halder et al. 2019; Palmer et al. 2020; Walther et al. 2013; Mozos et al. 2017)], osteoporosis and osteoarthritis (Schwalfenberg 2017; Simes et al. 2019; Azuma and Inoue 2019; Halder et al. 2019). In fact, a number of case-control studies suggested that vitamin K was associated with lower risk of osteoarthritis and could even potentially prevent it (activation of matrix Gla proteins by vitamin K could negatively regulate cartilage calcification) (Chin 2020). The anti-inflammatory role of vitamin K [via suppression of nuclear factor-κB (NK-κB) signal transduction] has also been reported [(Ciebiera et al. 2020; Shioi et al. 2020) and references therein]. Vitamin K is also implicated in mitigation of cognitive diseases (Simes et al. 2020; Schwalfenberg 2017). *In vivo* studies and human observational and interventional studies on glucose metabolism, diabetes and obesity have also identified another role for vitamin K (Bourron and Phan 2019; Schwalfenberg 2017).

Antitumor Role of Vitamin K

The anticancer functions of vitamin K had attracted attention relatively soon following its discovery, with increasing data in the last decades. Vitamin K antitumor effects have been examined in the following types of cancer: bladder (Di et al. 2017; Jiang et al. 2013), breast (Jiang et al. 2013; Di et al. 2017; Jamison et al. 2001; Dasari et al. 2017), cervical (Jamison et al. 2001), colon (Jiang et al. 2013; Jamison et al. 2001; Dasari et al. 2017), leukaemia (Jiang et al. 2013; Di et al. 2017; Jamison et al. 2001; Shibayama-Imazu et al. 2008; Dasari et al. 2017), liver (Ciebiera et al. 2020; Jamison et al. 2001; Shibayama-Imazu et al. 2008; Jiang et al. 2013; Di et al. 2017; Kaneki et al. 2006; Mizuta and Ozaki 2008; Dasari et al. 2017; Jinghe et al. 2015; Louka et al. 2017), lung (Jiang et al. 2013; Jinghe et al. 2015; Di et al. 2017; Jamison et al. 2001; Shibayama-Imazu et al. 2008; Schwalfenberg 2017; Dasari et al. 2017), nasopharyngeal (Jamison et al. 2001), oral (Jiang et al. 2013; Di et al. 2017; Dasari et al. 2017), ovarian (Shibayama-Imazu et al. 2008), pancreatic (Shibayama-Imazu et al. 2008; Schwalfenberg 2017; Davis-Yadley and Malafa 2015), prostate (Jinghe et al. 2015; Di et al. 2017; Schwalfenberg 2017; Dasari et al. 2017; Jiang et al. 2013), renal (Dasari et al. 2017), stomach (Jamison et al. 2001). Studies, including those reviewed in the aforementioned literature, have investigated how vitamin K could influence common tumour pathways and hence lead to suppression of cell growth, promotion of cell cycle arrest, induction of differentiation and apoptosis (Ivanova et al. 2018; Ciebiera et al. 2020; Mizuta and Ozaki 2008).

Antitumor Role of Vitamin K in Osteosarcoma and Possible Underlying Mechanisms of Action

Focus in the present chapter is on the anticancer effect of vitamin K and its analogs (all forms irrespectively) in osteosarcoma, with an emphasis on the signalling pathways that are activated following exposure to these compounds.

Osteosarcoma is the most common bone malignancy diagnosed in children and young adults. Although the overall 5 year survival rate of patients with osteosarcoma is approximately 60% and has tripled since the 1970s, prognosis for patients still remains unsatisfactory. Osteosarcoma is highly heterogeneous in its manifestation and characterized by resistance to chemotherapy and the development of metastases. Identification of agents that both inhibit tumour cell growth and metastatic activity, is deemed essential and timely (Czarnecka et al. 2020; Corre et al. 2020; Fan et al. 2020; de Azevedo et al. 2020).

Studies on the role of vitamin K in osteosarcoma cells are rather limited and mainly involve examination of the effect of menadione and of menadione-4 analogue (see Vitamin K: General Concepts). It is worth mentioning that menadione has been reported to cause adverse effects and show toxicity, and has been replaced from human consumption since 1963. Furthermore, at high concentrations, menadione is considered a cytotoxic substance which can undergo redox cycling, leading to oxidative stress-induced tissue injury. Specifically between 1980s and early 2000, menadione became one of the most popular chemicals known to induce cell death (Hallmann et al. 2004).

Menadione (5 and/or 10 μM) has been reported to inhibit viability and cause morphological changes such as cell shrinkage, induce DNA fragmentation and subsequently apoptosis in human MG-63 osteosarcoma cells (Wei et al. 2012). Menadione-induced apoptosis was caspase-dependent and this induction was associated with promotion of reactive oxygen species (ROS) production and reduction of mitochondrial membrane potential, indicative of the intrinsic apoptotic cell death signalling pathway (Wei et al. 2012). Special AT-rich sequence binding protein 2 (SATB2), a DNA-binding protein and regulator of gene expression, cell differentiation and survival, was shown to be up-regulated upon exposure to menadione (both mRNA and protein levels) (Wei et al. 2012). Both antiproliferative activity and apoptosis were shown to be further increased by silencing SATB2 (Wei et al. 2012). Interestingly, authors characterized the use of osteosarcoma MG-63 cells as a limitation to the study and in their attempt to evaluate the potential protective role of SATB2 in human osteoblasts (Wei et al. 2012).

In a number of studies performed in osteoblastoma cells, a research group attempted to identify key contributors and examined the mechanism responsible for the switch of cell death mode from apoptosis to necrosis. Studies were performed either in the 143B osteosarcoma cell line [containing mitochondrial DNA (mtDNA) and referred to as ρ^+) or in its mtDNA-less derivative (referred to as ρ^0). Regardless of the particularities in the findings [best summarized in (Wochna et al. 2007; Wochna et al. 2005; Kaminski et al. 2004)], all studies corroborated the fact that menadione (100 µM) inhibited viability of both osteosarcoma cells; inducing cell death either by apoptosis or necrosis, depending on the duration of menadione treatment. Exposure to menadione also increased ROS levels. NADPH oxidase inhibitors were shown to decrease menadione-induced ROS production and the inhibition of cell growth and/or switch to apoptotic/necrotic mode.

Menadione-4 (25, 35 µM) has been reported to inhibit viability (IC_{50} = 25 µM), induce morphological changes indicative of cell death, promote S phase cell cycle arrest and ultimately induce apoptosis of human U2OS osteosarcoma cells (Di et al. 2017). Furthermore, menadione-4 suppressed migration of U2OS cells (Di et al. 2017), a rather interesting outcome considering the fact that osteosarcoma is a metastatic type of cancer and that cell migration may be considered a surrogate for metastasis formation. Induction of apoptosis was associated with promotion of ROS generation and disruption of mitochondrial membrane potential, as was the case for menadione (Wei et al. 2012). Menadione-4 promoted caspase 3 cleavage and treatment of cells in the presence of the caspase inhibitor carbobenzoxy-valyl-alanyl-aspartyl-(O-methyl)-fluoromethylketone (Z-VAD-FMK), significantly inhibited the apoptotic effects of menadione-4. In addition, menadione-4 significantly decreased the expression of the anti apoptotic protein Bcl-2 and increased pro-apoptotic Bax protein expression (Di et al. 2017). Overall, menadione-4-induced apoptosis in U2OS cells has been suggested to be mediated through the mitochondrial pathway (intrinsic apoptosis) (Di et al. 2017).

Vitamin K2 (10^{-7}-10^{-5} M) and interestingly vitamin D3 (10^{-9}-10^{-7} mM), which will be discussed later, were found to inhibit MG-63 proliferation with the inhibitory effect of the latter being more pronounced (Zenmyo et al. 2001). Treatment with either vitamin K2 or vitamin D3 resulted in promotion of G0/G1 cell cycle arrest, which again was more pronounced in vitamin D3-treated MG-63 osteosarcoma cells (Zenmyo et al. 2001).

Vitamin K2 has also been shown to act as a transcriptional regulator of gene expression in osteosarcoma cells. Vitamin K2 has been reported to bind to and activate the steroid and xenobiotic receptor (SXR) in osteosarcoma cells and induce expression of its target gene CYP3A4 (Tabb et al. 2003).

VITAMIN D

Vitamin D: General Concepts

Vitamin D, the "sunshine vitamin," was also originally discovered approximately a century ago. As far as sources of vitamin D are concerned, >90% of the human requirement of vitamin D is synthesized in the skin from 7-dehydrocholesterol following exposure to sunlight, and the remaining is obtained from dietary sources.

Vitamin D is a family of lipid-soluble steroid compounds. The three main types of vitamin D are vitamin D1 (calciferol), vitamin D2 (ergocalciferol) and vitamin D3 (cholecalciferol). Vitamin D1 is found mostly in fish oils, vitamin D2 in plants and fungi and vitamin D3 is obtained from animal sources (Davis-Yadley and Malafa 2015; Ciebiera et al. 2020; Lanham-New 2008; Iijima et al. 2012).

Vitamin D is initially biologically inactive. Vitamin D is first transported via circulation to the liver, where it is activated to 25-hydroxycholecalciferol (calcidiol 25(OH)D, measure of circulating vitamin D in the blood, bound to vitamin D binding protein) (Louka et al. 2017; Davis-Yadley and Malafa 2015). It is then transported for further conversion in the kidney to form hormonally active 1-α,25-dihydroxycholecalciferol (1,25(OH)2D or 1-α,25(OH)2D or calcitriol) (Louka et al. 2017; Davis-

Yadley and Malafa 2015; Lanham-New 2008; Iijima et al. 2012). Interestingly, use of the active form of vitamin D3 is limited, as high concentrations have been shown to cause hypercalcemia and hypercalciuria (Yasuda et al. 2018).

Vitamin D: Functions

Vitamin D has been reported to maintain blood calcium homeostasis (Louka et al. 2017), regulate bone metabolism (Ciebiera et al. 2020) and stimulate bone maturation (Lanham-New 2008). Vitamin D has also been implicated in osteoarthritis, osteoporosis, diabetes mellitus, cardiovascular and autoimmune diseases (Kurucu et al. 2019). Reduced vitamin D levels have been identified in gynecological and obstetric pathologies, such as infertility, polycystic ovary syndrome and premature delivery (Ciebiera et al. 2020), as well as certain neurodegenerative conditions (Zayny et al. 2019).

Most of the biological functions of calcitriol are mediated through its nuclear receptor (VDR) (Zayny et al. 2019).

Antitumor Role of Vitamin D

Vitamin D antitumor effects have been examined in the following types of cancer: breast (Louka et al. 2017; Maayah et al. 2018), colorectal (Louka et al. 2017), liver (Louka et al. 2017), melanoma (Maayah et al. 2018), pancreatic (Davis-Yadley and Malafa 2015), prostate (Dasari et al. 2017; Louka et al. 2017). Readers interested in the topic are encouraged to read the aforementioned comprehensive literature/reviews and the references therein.

Antitumor Role of Vitamin D in Osteosarcoma and Possible Underlying Mechanisms of Action

Regarding the role of vitamin D in osteosarcoma, this chapter focused on literature published during the last 10 years and in particular on studies examining the effect of vitamin D, as a single agent or in combination, on human cell osteosarcoma proliferation and/or apoptosis, and not on VDR expression and its correlation with the progression of the disease. It has been noticed that vitamin D response is variable in different cancers, but even within different cell lines of the same type of cancer. This chapter focuses on human osteosarcoma cells, where response to vitamin D has been reported to be either positive or negative, hence reducing or not osteosarcoma proliferative ability.

Vitamin D was conjugated to doxorubicin (DOX-Vit D), in an attempt to overcome drug resistance and enhance delivery of the latter into cells (Maayah et al. 2018). DOX-Vit D (10 μM, but not DOX) was reported to suppress MG-63 cell proliferation (a response partially, but significantly, reversed by p38 and JNK inhibitors, suggesting a MAPK-dependent mechanism), and this antiproliferative effect was shown to be attributed to the up-regulation of caspase 3 and BCLxs mRNA expression. These proapoptotic genes were up-regulated via the involvement of both the extrinsic (increase of death receptor DR-4 mRNA expression) and intrinsic (increase of mRNA expression of the oxidative stress markers, NQO-1 and HO-1, and promotion of ROS production) apoptotic pathways and through the activation of MAPK signaling pathway (increased protein expression of p-JNK and p-p38, but not of p-Erk1/2), as well as inhibition of survival pathways (decrease of p-Akt and p-mTOR protein expression, no effect on binding activity of NF-κB) (Maayah et al. 2018).

Vitamin D (10 nM) has been found to inhibit proliferation of MG-63 (more pronounced effect) and Saos-2. Combination treatment consisting of vitamin D and genistein, a flavonoid exhibiting cancer preventive activity, was shown to reduce proliferation (induced by genistein) to control levels in both osteosarcoma cell lines (Engel et al. 2017). Combination treatment increased ERβ and VDR expression, mainly in MG-63. It also significantly decreased extracellular acidification and respiration rates in MG-63, which was however not fully supported by protein expression levels of key enzymes of the processes. Metabolic profiling and analysis upon combination treatment revealed up-regulation of ethanolamine, which was attributed to overexpression of the enzyme sphingosine-1-phosphate lyase (after combination treatment), which degrades sphingosine-1-phosphate, thus producing ethanolamine (Engel et al. 2017).

Suppression of proliferation of the human osteosarcoma lines U2OS, SJSA1, and Saos2 in response to calcitriol has been shown to be less pronounced compared to AXT cells, a relatively newly established mouse osteosarcoma cell line, and so was the promotion of G1 cell cycle arrest (Shimizu et al. 2017). Antiproliferative activity and inhibition of cell cycle progression, in AXT cells, was attributed to induction of endoplasmic reticulum (ER) stress manifested via down-regulation of cyclin D1 protein expression, increased p-p38 and p-Akt protein expression and promotion of ROS generation; it was reversed by silencing Atf4 and Ddit3, genes implicated in the ER stress response, and was not associated with vitamin D3 receptor protein expression (Shimizu et al. 2017). In human cells, calcitriol-induced DDIT3 mRNA expression was statistically increased in Saos2 and U2OS cells, but still more modestly, correlating with the weaker antiproliferative activity (Shimizu et al. 2017).

Vitamin D (100 nM) treatment of 143B osteosarcoma cells has revealed a plethora of differentially expressed genes regulating a diverse array of functions including inflammation, oxidative stress, bone mineral density, aggregation of bone cancer cells and more (Garimella et al. 2017). Analysis identified vitamin D-induced inhibition of the mRNA expression of Runx2, Runx2 target genes and vitamin D target genes. More importantly, vitamin D was shown to inhibit migration of osteosarcoma cells and even their invasion through matrigel, a functional effect of vitamin D in agreement with some of the identified genes from the microarray data (Garimella et al. 2017).

Vitamin D (100 nM) has been shown to inhibit MG-63 cell proliferation. Silencing of LIMK1 was shown to inhibit cell proliferation, which was not further inhibited upon vitamin D addition, suggestive of common pathways shared by LIMK1 and vitamin D, which mediate osteosarcoma growth inhibition. Vitamin D was shown to increase p-cofilin protein expression (Zhang et al. 2014).

Vitamin D (1000 nM) has been reported to inhibit Saos-2 proliferation, and this antiproliferative effect was enhanced upon silencing of Snail-1. Similarly, vitamin D was reported to induce apoptosis, which again was enhanced when Snail-1 was silenced. In the presence of vitamin D and upon silencing Snail-1, the rate of cell invasion was decreased (Yang et al. 2011). Silencing of Snail-1 in Saos-2 cells resulted in increased VDR protein expression. Upon treatment with vitamin D and silencing of Snail-1, β-catenin expression was found to be decreased, suggesting an important role for Snail-1/VDR/β-catenin axis on osteosarcoma progression. *In vitro* results were strengthened by *in vivo* observations in nude mice injected with either mock-infected or Snail-1 Saos-2 cells; mice injected with Snail-1-infected cells and treated with vitamin D showed inhibition of tumor growth. Furthermore, mRNA expression of β-catenin, c-Myc and cyclin D1 was decreased in tumor tissues (Yang et al. 2011).

Vitamin D has also been found not to affect proliferation of three osteosarcoma cell lines, namely MG-63, U2OS and Saos-2 (Matsugaki et al. 2010). Vitamin D, however, increased differentiation; it increased osteocalcin (OCN, as a marker of cell differentiation) production in MG-63 and U2OS cells. Vitamin D also increased N-myc downstream regulated gene 1 (NDRG1)/Cap43 expression in MG-63 and U2OS. Interestingly, the acquired invasiveness of Saos-2, correlated with decreased NDRG1/Cap43 expression. Furthermore, silencing of NDRG1/Cap43 in U2OS cells enhanced cell proliferation, suppressed p21 expression and OCN production (Matsugaki et al. 2010).

Vitamin D (1-1000 nM) and 25(OH)D3 were shown not to have an effect on Ki67 expression (a marker of proliferation) in Saos-2 and 143B osteosarcoma cells. Vitamin D (100 nM) was shown to decrease Saos-2 proliferation, while 143B cell proliferation was even increased upon exposure to 25(OH)D3 (100 nM) or vitamin D (10 nM) (Thompson et al. 2012). Treatment with vitamin D also significantly increased VDR expression in Saos-2 cells. Both vitamin D and 25(OH)D3 induced osteoblastic differentiation in both cell lines, as indicated by increases in alkaline phosphatase (ALP) activity, OCN mRNA expression, and mineralization. 25(OH)D3 induced apoptosis in both osteosarcoma cell lines, while vitamin D achieved this at higher concentrations. Both vitamin D and 25(OH)D3 increased the percentage of late stage apoptotic 143B cells (Thompson et al. 2012).

Link between Vitamin K and Vitamin D

After having introduced the two lipophilic vitamins and discussed their involvement in osteosarcoma, this section will highlight similarities and links between them.

Even 4 decades ago, it had been noted that vitamin K-dependent proteins' rate of synthesis was regulated and increased by vitamin D3 (Price and Baukol 1980; Fusaro et al. 2011). Hence, vitamin D has been shown to promote production of vitamin K-dependent proteins, which themselves require vitamin K for their carboxylation so as to function properly. Both vitamins K and D have been reported to play an important role in bone metabolism and immune function (Iijima et al. 2012), in calcium metabolism, in cardiovascular health (van Ballegooijen et al. 2017).

In vitro and *in vivo* studies, as well as clinical trials, nowadays, support more and more the notion of the synergistic effect of vitamin K combined with vitamin D in several physiological and pathological aspects such as bone health and metabolism [reviewed in (Simes et al. 2020; Tsugawa and Shiraki 2020; Lanham-New 2008, Weber 2001)] or cardiovascular-related conditions [reviewed in (van Ballegooijen et al. 2017; Kidd 2010; Mozos et al. 2017)].

CONCLUSION

In vitro evaluation of the role of vitamins K and D advocates for their importance in the progression of osteosarcoma. Unfortunately, to our knowledge, there are no active or completed clinical studies to date evaluating the role of either vitamin K or vitamin D in osteosarcoma treatment. Therefore, there is not yet enough available evidence from which to draw solid conclusions and clarify their role.

In the meantime, efforts are and should be concentrating on several avenues. Several vitamin K and D analogues have and are being synthesized to identify more potent compounds (Carr et al. 2002; Jinghe et al. 2015; Davis-Yadley and Malafa 2015). At the same time, many studies have been and should be currently evaluating antitumor activity of vitamins K and D and/or their analogues in combination with standard chemotherapeutics (Jinghe et al. 2015; Ciebiera et al. 2020). Interestingly, vitamin K and doxorubicin, a widely used chemotherapy drug, share a similarity, the quinone moiety. This fact further supports the belief that there is more than meets the eye regarding vitamin K (Dasari et al. 2017).

To summarize, vitamins K and D seem to affect crucial events during osteosarcoma tumorigenesis, such as proliferation, cell cycle progression, apoptosis, migration. This justifies the increasing interest in the elucidation of their role in bone tumors, and especially osteosarcoma.

REFERENCES

Akbari, S., and A. A. Rasouli-Ghahroudi. 2018. "Vitamin K and bone metabolism: A review of the latest evidence in preclinical studies." *Biomed Res Int*. doi: 10.1155/2018/4629383.

Azuma, K., and S. Inoue. 2019. "Multiple modes of vitamin K actions in aging-related musculoskeletal disorders." *Int J Mol Sci* 20. doi: 10.3390/ijms20112844.

Bourron, O., and F. Phan. 2019. "Vitamin K: A nutrient which plays a little-known role in glucose metabolism." *Curr Opin Clin Nutr Metab Care* 22:174-181. doi: 10.1097/MCO.0000000000000541.

Carr, B. I., Z. Wang, and S. Kar. 2002. "K vitamins, PTP antagonism, and cell growth arrest." *J Cell Physiol* 193:263-74. doi: 10.1002/jcp.10171.

Chin, K. Y. 2020. "The relationship between vitamin K and osteoarthritis: A review of current evidence." *Nutrients* 12. doi: 10.3390/nu12051208.

Ciebiera, M., M. Ali, M. Zgliczynska, M. Skrzypczak, and A. Al-Hendy. 2020. "Vitamins and uterine fibroids: current data on pathophysiology and possible clinical relevance." *Int J Mol Sci* 21. doi: 10.3390/ijms21155528.

Corre, I., F. Verrecchia, V. Crenn, F. Redini, and V. Trichet. 2020. "The osteosarcoma microenvironment: A complex but targetable ecosystem." *Cells* 9. doi: 10.3390/cells9040976.

Czarnecka, A. M., K. Synoradzki, W. Firlej, E. Bartnik, P. Sobczuk, M. Fiedorowicz, P. Grieb, and P. Rutkowski. 2020. "Molecular biology of osteosarcoma." *Cancers* (Basel) 12. doi: 10.3390/cancers12082130.

Dasari, S., S. M. Ali, G. Zheng, A. Chen, V. S. Dontaraju, M. C. Bosland, A. Kajdacsy-Balla, and G. Munirathinam. 2017. "Vitamin K and its analogs: potential avenues for prostate cancer management." *Oncotarget* 8:57782-57799. doi: 10.18632/oncotarget.17997.

Davis-Yadley, A. H., and M. P. Malafa. 2015. "Vitamins in pancreatic cancer: A review of underlying mechanisms and future applications." *Adv Nutr* 6:774-802. doi: 10.3945/an.115.009456.

de Azevedo, J. W. V., T. A. A. de Medeiros Fernandes, J. V. Fernandes, Jr., J. C. V. de Azevedo, D. C. F. Lanza, C. M. Bezerra, V. S. Andrade, J. M. G. de Araujo, and J. V. Fernandes. 2020. "Biology and pathogenesis of human osteosarcoma." *Oncol Lett* 19:1099-1116. doi: 10.3892/ol.2019.11229.

Di, W., M. Khan, Y. Gao, J. Cui, D. Wang, M. Qu, L. Feng, A. Maryam, and H. Gao. 2017. "Vitamin K4 inhibits the proliferation and induces apoptosis of U2OS osteosarcoma cells via mitochondrial dysfunction." *Mol Med Rep* 15:277-284. doi: 10.3892/mmr.2016.6001.

Engel, N., A. Adamus, N. Schauer, J. Kuhn, B. Nebe, G. Seitz, and K. Kraft. 2017. "Synergistic action of genistein and calcitriol in immature osteosarcoma MG-63 cells by SGPL1 up-regulation." *PLoS One* 12:e0169742. doi: 10.1371/journal.pone.0169742.

Fan, T. M., R. D. Roberts, and M. M. Lizardo. 2020. "Understanding and modeling metastasis biology to improve therapeutic strategies for combating osteosarcoma progression." *Front Oncol* 10:13. doi: 10.3389/fonc.2020.00013.

Fusaro, M., G. Crepaldi, S. Maggi, F. Galli, A. D'Angelo, L. Calo, S. Giannini, D. Miozzo, and M. Gallieni. 2011. "Vitamin K, bone fractures, and vascular calcifications in chronic kidney disease: An important but poorly studied relationship." *J Endocrinol Invest* 34:317-23. doi: 10.1007/BF03347093.

Garimella, R., P. Tadikonda, O. Tawfik, S. Gunewardena, P. Rowe, and P. Van Veldhuizen. 2017. "Vitamin D impacts the expression of Runx2 target genes and modulates inflammation, oxidative stress and membrane vesicle biogenesis gene networks in 143B osteosarcoma cells." *Int J Mol Sci* 18. doi: 10.3390/ijms18030642.

Halder, M., P. Petsophonsakul, A. C. Akbulut, A. Pavlic, F. Bohan, E. Anderson, K. Maresz, R. Kramann, and L. Schurgers. 2019. "Vitamin K: Double bonds beyond coagulation insights into differences between vitamin K1 and K2 in health and disease." *Int J Mol Sci* 20. doi: 10.3390/ijms20040896.

Hallmann, A., J. Klimek, M. Masaoka, M. Kaminski, J. Kedzior, A. Majczak, E. Niemczyk, M. Wozniak, P. Trzonkowski, and T. Wakabayashi. 2004. "Partial characterization of human choriocarcinoma cell line JAR cells in regard to oxidative stress." *Acta Biochim Pol* 51:1023-38.

Iijima, H., S. Shinzaki, and T. Takehara. 2012. "The importance of vitamins D and K for the bone health and immune function in inflammatory bowel disease." *Curr Opin Clin Nutr Metab Care* 15:635-40. doi: 10.1097/MCO.0b013e328357f623.

Ivanova, D., Z. Zhelev, P. Getsov, B. Nikolova, I. Aoki, T. Higashi, and R. Bakalova. 2018. "Vitamin K: Redox-modulation, prevention of mitochondrial dysfunction and anticancer effect." *Redox Biol* 16:352-358. doi: 10.1016/j.redox.2018.03.013.

Jamison, J. M., J. Gilloteaux, H. S. Taper, and J. L. Summers. 2001. "Evaluation of the *in vitro* and *in vivo* antitumor activities of vitamin C and K-3 combinations against human prostate cancer." *J Nutr* 131:158S-160S. doi: 10.1093/jn/131.1.158S.

Jiang, Y., J. Yang, C. Yang, F. Meng, Y. Zhou, B. Yu, M. Khan, and H. Yang. 2013. "Vitamin K4 induces tumor cytotoxicity in human prostate carcinoma PC-3 cells via the mitochondria-related apoptotic pathway." *Pharmazie* 68:442-8.

Jinghe, X., T. Mizuta, and I. Ozaki. 2015. "Vitamin K and hepatocellular carcinoma: the basic and clinic." *World J Clin Cases* 3:757-64. doi: 10.12998/wjcc.v3.i9.757.

Kaminski, M., E. Niemczyk, M. Masaoka, M. Karbowski, A. Hallmann, J. Kedzior, A. Majczak, D. Knap, Y. Nishizawa, J. Usukura, M. Wozniak, J. Klimek, and T. Wakabayashi. 2004. "The switch mechanism of the cell death mode from apoptosis to necrosis in menadione-treated human osteosarcoma cell line 143B cells." *Microsc Res Tech* 64:255-8. doi: 10.1002/jemt.20083.

Kaneki, M., T. Hosoi, Y. Ouchi, and H. Orimo. 2006. "Pleiotropic actions of vitamin K: Protector of bone health and beyond?." *Nutrition* 22:845-52. doi: 10.1016/j.nut.2006.05.003.

Kidd, P. M. 2010. "Vitamins D and K as pleiotropic nutrients: clinical importance to the skeletal and cardiovascular systems and preliminary evidence for synergy." *Altern Med Rev* 15:199-222.

Kurucu, N., G. Sahin, N. Sari, S. Ceylaner, and I. E. Ilhan. 2019. "Association of vitamin D receptor gene polymorphisms with osteosarcoma risk and prognosis." *J Bone Oncol* 14:100208. doi: 10.1016/j.jbo.2018.100208.

Lanham-New, S. A. 2008. "Importance of calcium, vitamin D and vitamin K for osteoporosis prevention and treatment." *Proc Nutr Soc* 67:163-76. doi: 10.1017/S0029665108007003.

Louka, M. L., A. M. Fawzy, A. M. Naiem, M. F. Elseknedy, A. E. Abdelhalim, and M. A. Abdelghany. 2017. "Vitamin D and K signaling pathways in hepatocellular carcinoma." *Gene* 629:108-116. doi: 10.1016/j.gene.2017.07.074.

Maayah, Z. H., T. Zhang, M. L. Forrest, S. Alrushaid, M. R. Doschak, N. M. Davies, and A. O. S. El-Kadi. 2018. "DOX-Vit D, a novel doxorubicin delivery approach, inhibits human osteosarcoma cell proliferation by inducing apoptosis while inhibiting Akt and mTOR signaling pathways." *Pharmaceutics* 10. doi: 10.3390/pharmaceutics10030144.

Marchili, M. R., E. Santoro, A. Marchesi, S. Bianchi, L. Rotondi Aufiero, and A. Villani. 2018. "Vitamin K deficiency: A case report and review of current guidelines." *Ital J Pediatr* 44:36. doi: 10.1186/s13052-018-0474-0.

Matsugaki, T., M. Zenmyo, K. Hiraoka, N. Fukushima, T. Shoda, S. Komiya, M. Ono, M. Kuwano, and K. Nagata. 2010. "N-myc downstream-regulated gene 1/Cap43 expression promotes cell differentiation of human osteosarcoma cells." *Oncol Rep* 24:721-5. doi: 10.3892/or_00000913.

Mizuta, T., and I. Ozaki. 2008. "Hepatocellular carcinoma and vitamin K." *Vitam Horm* 78:435-42. doi: 10.1016/S0083-6729(07)00018-0.

Mozos, I., D. Stoian, and C. T. Luca. 2017. "Crosstalk between vitamins A, B12, D, K, C, and E status and arterial stiffness." *Dis Markers* 2017:8784971. doi: 10.1155/2017/8784971.

Palmer, C. R., L. C. Blekkenhorst, J. R. Lewis, N. C. Ward, C. J. Schultz, J. M. Hodgson, K. D. Croft, and M. Sim. 2020. "Quantifying dietary vitamin K and its link to cardiovascular health: A narrative review." *Food Funct* 11:2826-2837. doi: 10.1039/c9fo02321f.

Price, P. A., and S. A. Baukol. 1980. "1,25-Dihydroxyvitamin D3 increases synthesis of the vitamin K-dependent bone protein by osteosarcoma cells." *J Biol Chem* 255:11660-3.

Rodriguez-Olleros Rodriguez, C., and M. Diaz Curiel. 2019. "Vitamin K and bone health: A review on the effects of vitamin K deficiency and supplementation and the effect of non-vitamin K antagonist oral anticoagulants on different bone parameters." *J Osteoporos* 2019:2069176. doi: 10.1155/2019/2069176.

Sato, T., L. J. Schurgers, and K. Uenishi. 2012. "Comparison of menaquinone-4 and menaquinone-7 bioavailability in healthy women." *Nutr J* 11:93. doi: 10.1186/1475-2891-11-93.

Schwalfenberg, G. K. 2017. "Vitamins K1 and K2: the emerging group of vitamins required for human health." *J Nutr Metab* 2017:6254836. doi: 10.1155/2017/6254836.

Shibayama-Imazu, T., T. Aiuchi, and K. Nakaya. 2008. "Vitamin K2-mediated apoptosis in cancer cells: role of mitochondrial transmembrane potential." *Vitam Horm* 78:211-26. doi: 10.1016/S0083-6729(07)00010-6.

Shimizu, T., W. A. Kamel, S. Yamaguchi-Iwai, Y. Fukuchi, A. Muto, and H. Saya. 2017. "Calcitriol exerts an anti-tumor effect in osteosarcoma by inducing the endoplasmic reticulum stress response." *Cancer Sci* 108:1793-1802. doi: 10.1111/cas.13304.

Shioi, A., T. Morioka, T. Shoji, and M. Emoto. 2020. "The inhibitory roles of vitamin K in progression of vascular calcification." *Nutrients* 12. doi: 10.3390/nu12020583.

Simes, D. C., C. S. B. Viegas, N. Araujo, and C. Marreiros. 2019. "Vitamin K as a powerful micronutrient in aging and age-related diseases: Pros and cons from clinical studies." *Int J Mol Sci* 20. doi: 10.3390/ijms20174150.

Simes, D. C., C. S. B. Viegas, N. Araujo, and C. Marreiros. 2020. "Vitamin K as a diet supplement with impact in human health: Current evidence in age-related diseases." *Nutrients* 12. doi: 10.3390/ nu12010138.

Tabb, M. M., A. Sun, C. Zhou, F. Grun, J. Errandi, K. Romero, H. Pham, S. Inoue, S. Mallick, M. Lin, B. M. Forman, and B. Blumberg. 2003. "Vitamin K2 regulation of bone homeostasis is mediated by the steroid and xenobiotic receptor SXR." *J Biol Chem* 278:43919-27. doi: 10.1074/jbc.M303136200.

Thompson, L., S. Wang, O. Tawfik, K. Templeton, J. Tancabelic, D. Pinson, H. C. Anderson, J. Keighley, and R. Garimella. 2012. "Effect of 25-hydroxyvitamin D3 and 1 α,25 dihydroxyvitamin D3 on differentiation and apoptosis of human osteosarcoma cell lines." *J Orthop Res* 30:831-44. doi: 10.1002/jor.21585.

Tsugawa, N., and M. Shiraki. 2020. "Vitamin K nutrition and bone health." *Nutrients* 12. doi: 10.3390/nu12071909.

van Ballegooijen, A. J., S. Pilz, A. Tomaschitz, M. R. Grubler, and N. Verheyen. 2017. "The synergistic interplay between vitamins D and K for bone and cardiovascular health: A narrative review." *Int J Endocrinol* 2017:7454376. doi: 10.1155/2017/7454376.

Walther, B., J. P. Karl, S. L. Booth, and P. Boyaval. 2013. "Menaquinones, bacteria, and the food supply: the relevance of dairy and fermented food products to vitamin K requirements." *Adv Nutr* 4:463-73. doi: 10.3945/an.113.003855.

Weber, P. 2001. "Vitamin K and bone health." *Nutrition* 17:880-7. doi: 10.1016/s0899-9007(01)00709-2.

Wei, J. D., Y. L. Lin, C. H. Tsai, H. S. Shieh, P. I. Lin, W. P. Ho, and R. M. Chen. 2012. "SATB2 participates in regulation of menadione-induced apoptotic insults to osteoblasts." *J Orthop Res* 30:1058-66. doi: 10.1002/jor.22046.

Wochna, A., E. Niemczyk, C. Kurono, M. Masaoka, J. Kedzior, E. Slominska, M. Lipinski, and T. Wakabayashi. 2007. "A possible role of oxidative stress in the switch mechanism of the cell death mode from apoptosis to necrosis-studies on ρ^0 cells." *Mitochondrion* 7:119-24. doi: 10.1016/j.mito.2006.11.005.

Wochna, A., E. Niemczyk, C. Kurono, M. Masaoka, A. Majczak, J. Kedzior, E. Slominska, M. Lipinski, and T. Wakabayashi. 2005. "Role of mitochondria in the switch mechanism of the cell death mode from apoptosis to necrosis-Studies on ρ^0 cells." *J Electron Microsc* (Tokyo) 54:127-38. doi: 10.1093/jmicro/dfi031.

Yang, H., Y. Zhang, Z. Zhou, X. Jiang, and A. Shen. 2011. "Snail-1 regulates VDR signaling and inhibits 1,25(OH)-D3 action in osteosarcoma." *Eur J Pharmacol* 670:341-6. doi: 10.1016/j.ejphar.2011.09.160.

Yasuda, K., E. Tohyama, M. Takano, A. Kittaka, M. Ohta, S. Ikushiro, and T. Sakaki. 2018. "Metabolism of 2α-[2-(tetrazol-2-yl)ethyl]-1α,25-dihydroxyvitamin D3 by CYP24A1 and biological activity of its 24R-hydroxylated metabolite." *J Steroid Biochem Mol Biol* 178:333-339. doi: 10.1016/j.jsbmb.2018.02.001.

Zayny, A., M. Almokhtar, K. Wikvall, O. Ljunggren, K. Ubhayasekera, J. Bergquist, P. Kibar, and M. Norlin. 2019. "Effects of glucocorticoids on vitamin D3-metabolizing 24-hydroxylase (CYP24A1) in Saos-2 cells and primary human osteoblasts." *Mol Cell Endocrinol* 496:110525. doi: 10.1016/j.mce.2019.110525.

Zenmyo, M., S. Komiya, T. Hamada, K. Hiraoka, S. Kato, T. Fujii, H. Yano, K. Irie, and K. Nagata. 2001. "Transcriptional activation of p21 by vitamin D3 or vitamin K2 leads to differentiation of p53-deficient MG-63 osteosarcoma cells." *Hum Pathol* 32:410-6. doi: 10.1053/hupa.2001.23524.

Zhang, H. S., J. W. Zhao, H. Wang, H. Y. Zhang, Q. Y. Ji, L. J. Meng, F. J. Xing, S. T. Yang, and Y. Wang. 2014. "LIM kinase 1 is required for insulin-dependent cell growth of osteosarcoma cell lines." *Mol Med Rep* 9:103-8. doi: 10.3892/mmr.2013.1798.

In: Vitamin Deficiency
Editors: N. Stewart and D. Thomson © 2021 Nova Science Publishers, Inc.
ISBN: 978-1-53618-979-7

Chapter 3

IMPLICATION OF VITAMIN K IN BONE HOMEOSTASIS AND OSSEOUS METABOLISM

Angelos Kaspiris[1,*,#]*, MD, MSc, PhD,*
Efstathios Chronopoulos[2,#]*, MD, PhD*
Evangelia Pantazaka[3]*, MSc, PhD,*
Olga D. Savvidou[4]*, MD, PhD,*
Elias Vasiliadis[5]*, MD, PhD*
and Elias Panagiotopoulos[6]*, MD, PhD*

[1]Laboratory of Molecular Pharmacology, Section of Orthopaedic Research, School of Health Sciences, University of Patras, Patras, Greece
[2]Second Orthopaedic Department, "Agia Olga" University Hospital and Medical School, National and Kapodistrian University of Athens, Greece
[3]Section of Organic Chemistry and Biochemistry, Department of Chemistry, University of Patras, Patras, Greece
[4]First Department of Orthopaedic Surgery, "ATTIKON" University Hospital and Medical School, National and Kapodistrian

---

* Corresponding Author's E-mail: angkaspiris@hotmail.com.
# Both authors have equally contributed to this chapter.

University of Athens, Athens, Greece
[5]Third Department of Orthopaedic Surgery, "KAT" University Hospital and Medical School, National and Kapodistrian University of Athens, Greece
[6]Orthopaedic Department, "Rion" University Hospital and Medical School, School of Health Sciences, University of Patras, Greece

ABSTRACT

Vitamin K (VK) is a fat-soluble multifunctional vitamin that was originally implicated in blood coagulation. However, current studies elucidate its pivotal role in the maintenance of bone strength, and its positive impact on bone metabolism. VK exerts its anabolic effects on the bone turnover by promoting osteoblast differentiation, by upregulating transcription of specific genes in osteoblasts, and by activating the bone-linked VK dependent proteins that are involved in the mineralization of extracellular bone matrix. Additionally, in vitro studies supported the effects of VK on the differentiation of other mesenchymal stem cells into osteoblasts. Similarly, in vivo experimental studies demonstrated that Steroid and Xenobiotic Receptor (SXR), a putative receptor for vitamin K, is important in the bone homeostasis and metabolism. Several epidemiological surveys revealed that VK status is associated with aging-related musculoskeletal diseases such as osteoporosis, osteoarthritis, and sarcopenia while the combination of vitamin VK and PTH increased the differentiation of osteoblasts appearing synergistic effects on bone formation of bone defects. Furthermore, low VK concentration in the serum was correlated with inflammation and low areal bone mineral density (aBMD) contributing to increased risk of incident fractures. The purpose of this chapter was to highlight the VK-depended biological pathways which are associated to the prevention and treatment of bone metabolism disorders.

Keywords: vitamin K, bone metabolism, bone mineral densisty, osteoblasts

INTRODUCTION

Bone is a metabolically active tissue that continually remodels itself in order to adjust to growth changes, to mechanical loads, to homeostasis alterations and to regulation of the bone marrow micro-environment. In the mature skeleton, bone remodeling provides calcium and phosphate systemically and replaces aged or damaged bone maintaining bone health [1, 2]. When hard tissue dispoportion between resorption and formation of hard tissue develops, bone homeostasis deteriorates. Increased bone resorption is associated with weak bones and an elevated risk of fractures. This characteristic was observed in several bone diseases like osteoporosis, hyperparathyroidism, renal osteodystrophy, Paget's disease and metastatic bone disease [3]. Despite the fact that the loss of bone mass and the deterioration of the internal bone structure is affected by genetic and physiological factors like age, sex, ethnicity or medication use, lifestyle and nutritional factors, such as tobacco use or alcohol consumption, low activity levels or inadequate sun exposure, the poor intake of vitamins and minerals is also implicated in the development of low Bone Mineral Density (BMD) [4]. It has been suggested that vitamin K, initially known for its effect on blood coagulation, is involved in musculoskeletal metabolism. Vitamin K refers to a group of fat-soluble compounds. There are several vitamin K-dependent proteins involved in coagulation, bone development, and cardiovascular health. Vitamin K deficiency was correlated with significant bleeding, poor bone development, osteoporosis, and increased cardiovascular disease [5]. According to the National Academy of Science Food and Nutrition Board, the dietary requirements of healthy adults is 120 and 90 µg/day for men and women, respectively [6].

Vitamin K Deficiency Bleeding (VKDB) in newborns can be classified into three categories based on the timing of the presentation. Early VKDB presents within 24 hours after birth, classic VKDB presents within the first week, and late VKDB presents between one to twelve weeks of life.

VITAMIN K

Vitamin K: General Concepts

Vitamin K is a family of fat-soluble compounds that share a 2-methyl-1, 4-naphthoquinone structure called menadione and a side chain at the 3-

position [5, 7]. Based on the location of the side chain, three main types of vitamin K, have been classified as: Vitamin K1 (phylloquinone), Vitamin K2 (menaquinones) and Vitamin K3 (menadione). Among them, vitamins K1 and K2 are natural compounds while vitamin K3 is artificial.

Vitamin K1 is formed by a phytyl side chain, and it constitutes the main dietary source of vitamin K in the Western population [5, 7]. It is synthesized by plants and cyanobacteria, and it can be found in green leafy vegetables and fruits (kiwifruit, avocado, broccoli, green grapes, and lettuce), in vegetable-derived oils (canola, soybean, and olive oil), and in grains [5, 7].

Vitamin K2 is formed by a polymeric side chain of repeating prenyl units and is synthesized by certain bacteria. Vitamin K2 is classified into 13 subtypes (MK-2 to MK-14) according to the number of prenyl units. The majority of prenyl units are unsaturated, but some bacteria produce saturated units, adding extra hydrogen atoms to the MK subtype. Vitamin K2 subtypes are synthesized by anaerobic bacteria of the human colon (except MK-4) [5, 7] or by food bacteria such as animal liver and fermented foods. Long-chain vitamin K2 is produced by enteric flora and has low bioactivity. MK-4, which is produced from vitamin K2 in a two-phase process by the conversion of menadione in specific tissues such as testes, pancreas, and vessel wall, is the predominant form of vitamin K in human body and it can be found in fish, liver, milk, vegetables and eggs.

Vitamin K3 or menadione is a water-soluble type of vitamin K lacking a side chain. Additionally, it is a synthetic analog added to animal food and it is converted to MK-4 in the liver. It has also been reported that several long chain vitamin K2 subtypes can be converted to MK-4 [5, 7].

Vitamin K is absorbed by the small intestine and it is transferred to the liver and other tissues through the lymphatic system. The larger amount of vitamin K1 is accumulated in the liver and the rest which is linked to vitamin K2 is allocated to other tissues by the low density lipoproteins. Vitamin K1 and long-chain forms of vitamin K2 are stored mainly in liver, but vitamin K2 (in the form of MK 4) is also stored in glands, like pancreas and in genital organs. Therefore, deficiency of vitamin K may increase the risk of cancers, of cardiovascular disease, of soft tissue calcification, or osteoporosis through physiological pathways that affect specific organs [5, 7-13].

Vitamin K: Mechanisms of Action

Four major mechanisms have been reported concerning the role of Vitamin K in the osseous metabolism.

According yo first mechanism, which is the most known, vitamin K carboxylates glutamic acid (Glu) residues that are located in vitamin K-dependent proteins and acts as coenzyme for the gamma-glutamyl carboxylase (GGCX) enzyme converting them into gamma-carboxyglutamic acid (Gla), adding a carboxyl group to gamma-position carbon of glutamate residues [7, 14].

Many bone vitamin K-dependent proteins have been detected and such as:

1. Matrix Gla protein, which is expressed in osteoblasts and regulates the calcification of bony tissues [7, 14-16],
2. Periostin, which is expressed in periosteum and regulates the development and maintenance of bones [7, 14, 17],
3. Growth Arrest Specific-6 (GAS-6), which is expressed in bone marrow cells, osteoblasts, osteoclasts and regulates the proliferation of osseous cells and increases the osteoclast activity [7, 14, 18]
4. Protein S, which increases the osteoclast activity [7, 14, 18]
5. TGFβ-induced (TGFBI) protein, which is expressed in bone and joint tissues and regulates the development and maintenance of bones [7, 14, 19]
6. Gla-rich protein/Upper zone of growth plate and Cartilage Matrix Associated (UCMA) protein, which is expressed in cartilage tissues and in chondrocytes as well as in osteoblasts and osteocytes regulating the calcification of the joint tissues [7, 14, 20-22]
7. γ-Gluatmyl Carboxylase (GGCX) [7, 14, 20] and
8. Osteocalcin (or Bone Gla protein), which is expressed in osteoblasts and regulates the calcification of bones [7, 14, 24-26]. In specific, during the bone mineralization phase, osteocalcin is secreted by the osteoblastic cells, and it is joined to calcium ions and to hydroxyapatite crystals [7, 24-26]. Osteocalcin contains three Glu

residues, and its binding capacity is correlated with its carboxylation degree. Serum levels of the undercarboxylated form of osteocalcin (ucOC) are positevely correlated with fracture risk and are used as biomarkers for vitamin K administration for the treatment of patients with vitamin K deficiency [14]. Moreover, osteocalcin is implicated in the regulation of energy metabolism leading to the conclusion that bone may in fact has a significant endocrine function [7, 24-26].

A second mechanism of action of vitamin K, is through the regulation of transcription of osteoblastic markers and the production of osteoclasts, altering the levels of bone resorption, as it was reported by *in vitro* studies [7, 27].

The third mechanism of action of vitamin K is caried out via the activation of the orphan nuclear Steroid and Xenobiotic Receptor (SXR) by Vitamin K2. In specific, the MK-4 form of vitamin K2 is a ligand of SXR receptor [7, 14, 28-29]. When a ligand binds to SXR receptor, a pathway is activated that leads to the expression of SXR target genes, like the drug metabolizing enzyme CYP3A4 or the ABC family transporter MDR1, which play important role in body detoxification and drug excretion [7, 14, 28-29]. Furthermore, SXR expression was detected in osteoblastic cells and was activated by the MK-4 form resulting in increased formation of bony tissue [4, 7, 30]. Nevertheless, we must underline the fact that vitamin K1 has not been reported to activate the SXR receptor leading to the assumption that the *in vivo* transformation of vitamin K1 to the MK-4 form was necessary in order to activate the osteoblasts through SXR binding [7, 14, 31].

Additionally, the finding that vitamin K2 interacted with 17β-Hydroxysteroid dehydrogenase type 4 (17β-HSD4), which is an enzyme implicated in estrogen signaling that converted estradiol to estrone, may explain the beneficial effects of MK-4 to musculoskeletal homeostasis [14, 32]. Finally, Karasawa et al., showed that the epoxide form of MK-4 modified the pro-apoptotic protein Bcl-2 antagonist killer 1 *(Bak)*, after forming covalent bonds at cysteine 166 [14, 33] This modification of *Bak* resulted in the induction of apoptosis in human promyelocytic cell HL60

[14, 33]. *Bak*, also, controlled the apoptotic procedure in osteoblastic cells. Similarly, it has been reported that the genetic deletion of *Bak* and *Bax* in osteoblastic cells, resulted in reduction of bone cell population apoptosis and in increased femoral cancellous bone mass and cortical porosity in aged mice [14, 34], suggesting that the covalent adjustment of *Bak* by MK-4, was implicated in skeletal metabolism.

Vitamin K, Osteoporosis and Fractures

Many studies have demonstrated that the combination of low concentration of K1 in the serum, with the elevated levels of undercarboxylated osteocalcin (ucOC), and the reduced intake of vitamins K1 and K2 were linked to increased risk of fractures [7]. However, the impact of vitamin K intake on BMD is still under investigation [7]. In the study of Jaghsi et al. [35], K1 serum levels were positively associated with BMD at the lumbar spine in postmenopausal women who did not receive any estrogen replacement medication [7, 28] suggesting that serum levels of vitamin K1 could be used as a reliable diagnostic marker of osteoporosis. However, rich diet in vitamin K may also be accompanied by other nutritional elements, such as calcium, magnesium, phosphorus that were implicated in bone metabolism [7] making the above findings ambiguous. In the study of Evenepoel et al, poor vitamin K status was correlated with inflammation and low BMD in End-Stage Renal Disease patients, but strong association between vitamin K status and bone turnover markers, like biointact PTH and FGF23, sclerostin, calcidiol, calcitriol or P1NP, BsAP, and TRAP5B, and dephosphorylated-uncarboxylated Matrix Gla Protein, was not observed [36].

Meta-analysis data from Fang et al. study revealed that, although supplementation of vitamin K did not affect BMD at the femoral neck remarkably, BMD at the lumbar spine was increased [37]. Regarding the form of the administered Vitamin K, data of the above study showed that vitamin K2 was very effective on BMD maintanance compared with vitamin K1 [37]. Extra subgroup analysis of the study detected that the changes were apparent only in Asian population and in non-postmenopausal women [37]. Similarly, meta-analysis of Huang et al. demonstrated that K2 supplements improved significantly the vertebral and forearm BMD in postmenopausal women with osteoporosis, supporting the hypothesis that vitamin K2 plays significant role not only in the maintenance and in improvement of vertebral BMD but also in the prevention of fractures in those patients [38]. In the recent meta-analysis by Mott et al, that was designed to assess the effectiveness of oral vitamin K supplementation in increasing bone mineral density and in reducing fracture rate in postmenopausal and osteoporotic patients, the analysis of 36 included studies showed that there was no sufficient evidence to confirm the positive correlation between vitamin K status and BMD or vertebral fractures [39]. Nevertheless, the frequency of clinical fractures was significantly lower in the vitamin K group of patients [39].

Latest research studies insisted on the positive relationship between circulating vitamin K1 concentrations with fracture risk and BMD. Specifically, results of the study of Moor et al. that analyzed the association between circulating levels of vitamin K1 with fracture risk as well as with BMD, hip geometry, plasma dephospho-uncarboxylated- Matrix Gla Protein (dp-ucMGP) and extra-hepatic vitamin K dependent protein (VKDP) in 374 postmenopausal women [40] showed that serum levels of vitamin K1 were significantly lower in the group with osteoporotic fractures and were independently associated with fracture risk [40]. Furthermore, serum vitamin K1 was positively correlated to cross-sectional area, to cross sectional moment of inertia and to section modulus at the narrow neck of femur, suggesting that the positive effect of vitamin K on fracture risk may be related to its effects on bone strength [40]. The authors proposed that higher concentrations of serum vitamin K1 may be required for vitamin K's skeletal effects compared to coagulation [40]. These results were in agreement with several *in vitro* and *in vivo* research studies. The concurrent administration of MK-4 and PTH for 8 weeks promoted bone formation and vascular formation in calvarial bone defects in osteopenic rats compared to control increasing serum level of Gla-OC [41]. Similarly, combined treatment with vitamin K2 and PTH showed positive effects on the prevention of bone loss in the femurs of ovariectomized Sprague Dawley rats. Moreover, the combined treatment was followed by increased serum Gla-OC and promoted bone formation in osteoporotic calvarial bone defects [42]. Additionally, immunohistochemical analysis showed that serum γ-carboxylated osteocalcin and RUNX2 were more highly expressed in the Vitamin K and PTH group than in the control group [42]. In the same study, *in vitro* results demonstrated that culture and treatment of the bone marrow-derived stem cells with PTH and vitamin K2, increased the expression of ALP, BMP2 and RUNX2 [42]. These data suggested that the combination of vitamin K2 and PTH increased the differentiation of osteoblasts and had a synergistic effect on bone formation in osteoporotic calvarial bone defects [42]. Another *in vivo study* showed that prior administration of vitamin K2 improves the therapeutic effects of zoledronic acid in ovariectomized rats and partially prevented the inhibition of bone formation caused by zoledronic acid as it was reflected by the indices of BMD, bone calcium content and bone strength [43]. The *in vitro* results of the same study demonstrated that the underlying mechanisms for the protective action of vitamin K2 pretreatment was due to the inhibition of apoptosis and the depression of sclerostin (Sost) expression in osteoblasts, which in turn led to the improvement of the therapeutic effects of zoledronic acid. These findings suggested that pretreatment administration of vitamin K2 might serve a new long-term therapy protocol for osteoporosis [43]. The above results may be also related to the protective effects of Vitamin K1 and K2 compounds on the proteomic profile of human osteoblasts under oxidative conditions induced by hydrogen peroxide (H_2O_2) enhancing the ability of bony tissues formation, remodeling, and mineralization [44].

Furthermore, the study by Knapen et al., [38] investigated the effects on the bone structure after the administration of low-dose vitamin K2 supplements (MK-7) and placebo for three years, in 244 healthy postmenopausal women. It was observed that increased MK-7 intake significantly improved vitamin K serum status and decreased the age-related decline in BMC and BMD at the lumbar spine and femoral neck, but not at the total hip. Bone strength (measured as compression, bending, and impact strength) was also strongly affected by MK-7. MK-7 significantly decreased the loss in vertebral height of the lower thoracic region at the mid-site of the vertebrae [45]. Regarding the implication of vitamin K in fracture pathophysiology, the systematic review and meta-analysis of Cockayne et al, investigated the association between both BMD and fracture risk after the administration of vitamin K1 or MK-4 supplements [46]. This systematic review analysed data of bone loss and fractures from thirteen and seven surveys respectively. All studies, but one, showed an advantage of Vitamin K1 and K2 in reducing of the bone loss suggesting that the supplementation with Vitamin K1 and MK-4was crucial for the restriction of bone defects. Interestingly, the analysis of fracture data, that concerned mainly Japanese postmenopausal women, revealed a reduced frequency of all fracture types in the patients who received MK-4 supplements [46]. However, a latest meta-analysis of observational studies, indicated that the use of vitamin K antagonists like warfarin was not associated with an increased risk for hip fracture, but it was correlated with raised rate of fractures in older and female patients [47], suggesting that the application of non-vitamin K antagonist oral anticoagulants (NOACs) may be a safer choice in elderly osteoporotic female patients with physical inactivity [48].

Roles of Vitamin K on Osteoarthritis and Sarcopenia

The relationship between vitamin K status and occurrence or progression of Osteoarthritis has been addressed in several studies [14, 49-52] indicating that vitamin K may prevent cartilage from degenerative changes. In the Framingham Offspring Study a negative relationship between the occurrence of hand OA, large osteophyte and joint space narrowing and circulating Vitamin K1 was found [51]. In addition, knee OA was not significantly associated with circulating Vitamin K1 in this study [51]. Similarly, in the Health Aging and Body Composition Study (Health ABC) study involving 791 community-dwelling elderly, a higher plasma uncarboxylated MGP level was associated with the occurrence of meniscus damage, osteophytes, bone marrow lesions, and subchonral bone cysts, but not with knee pain. Subgroup analysis based on race showed that, low uncarboxylated MGP was associated with articular cartilage damage in African Americans, while extremely low plasma vitamin K was associated with meniscal damage, in Caucasians [52]. In the clinical trial by Neogi et al., [53], the administration of 500 μg Vitamin K1 for 3 years did not alter the occurrence of hand OA, joint space narrowing, and osteophytes. Subgroup analysis reported that patients with vitamin K baseline insufficiency ($\leq$ 1nM), who achieved sufficiency after treatment, showed significant reduction in the occurrence of joint space narrowing, but not in radiographic OA and osteophytes. However, as both the treatment and control group had also received vitamin D supplementation, which helps prevent OA, the above results were questionable [53].

Despite the fact that the exact mechanism is not yet elucidated, it has been proposed that vitamin K protected the articular cartilage proteins from abnormal γ-carboxylation that it was involved in the aberrant calcification of cartilage [14]. Another molecule, which is involved in the cartilage protective effect of vitamin K, was Gla-rich protein (GRP). In osteoarthritic cartilage undercarboxylated GRP was more abundant than carboxylated GRP and both were associated with ectopic calcification [54]. This observation suggested that the γ-carboxylation of GRP played a key role in the inhibition of cartilage calcification [14].

Many clinical studies concluded that vitamin K status was related to physical performance. In the longitudinal cohort study study of van Ballegooijen et al, association between vitamin K status and physical functioning of 633 community-dwelling adults for over 13 years was examined. The plasma desphospho-uncarboxylated matrix Gla protein (dp-ucMGP) was measured as biomarker of vitamin K status. The outcome was obtained by the calculation of handgrip strength, of calf circumference, of self-reported functional limitations and of functional performance. In those patients the highest dp-ucMGP tertile was associated with lower handgrip strength, smaller calf circumference, and, only among women, poorer functional performance score, indicating that low vitamin K status may also be a potential reason for sarcopenic dysfunctional alterations [55]. Based on the above mentioned results, vitamin K seems to have beneficial effects on muscle quality and mass as it improved the physical performance scores [14].

CONCLUSION

Vitamin K plays a key role in bone health and is implicated in cartilage and bone metabolic pathways. Many research and clinical studies highlighted the fact that low vitamin K diet intake, low serum vitamin K levels, and increased plasma concentrations of ucOC are directly linked to increased risk of various types of fractures (especially hip fracture). However, the up to date results of the clinical surveys and meta-analyses did not allow us to draw definite conclusions. Future high-quality clinical trials are deemed necessary to clarify the exact role of vitamin K in the bone metabolic and musculoskeletal degenerative diseases.

REFERENCES

[1] Seeman E. Bone modeling and remodeling. *Crit. Rev. Eukaryot. Gene Expr.* 2009; 19: 219–233.

[2] Eriksen EF. Cellular mechanisms of bone remodeling. *Rev. Endocr. Metab. Disord.* 2010; 11: 219–227.

[3] Cummings SR, Melton LJ. Epidemiology and outcomes of osteoporotic fractures. *Lancet* 2002; 359: 1761–1767.

[4] Pouresmaeili F, Dehghan BK, Kamarehei M, Goh YM. A comprehensive overview on osteoporosis and its risk factors. *Ther. Clin. Risk Manag.* 2018; 14: 2029–2049.

[5] Akbari S, Rasouli-Ghahroudi AA. Vitamin K and Bone Metabolism: A Review of the Latest Evidence in Preclinical Studies. *Biomed. Res. Int.* 2018; 2018: 4629383.

[6] Shearer MJ, Fu X, Booth SL. Vitamin K nutrition, metabolism, and requirements: current concepts and future research. *Adv. Nutr.* 2012; 3(2): 182-195.

[7] Rodríguez-Olleros Rodríguez C, Díaz Curiel M. Vitamin K and Bone Health: A Review on the Effects of Vitamin K Deficiency and Supplementation and the Effect of Non-Vitamin K Antagonist Oral Anticoagulants on Different Bone Parameters. *J. Osteoporos.* 2019; 2019: 2069176.

[8] Orlando A, Linsalata M, Tutino V, D'Attoma B, Notarnicola M, Russo F. Vitamin K1 exerts antiproliferative effects and induces apoptosis in three differently graded human colon cancer cell lines. *Biomed. Res. Int.* 2015; 2015: 296721.

[9] Linsalata M, Orlando A, Tutino V, Notarnicola M, D'Attoma B, Russo F. Inhibitory effect of vitamin K1 on growth and polyamine biosynthesis of human gastric and colon carcinoma cell lines. *Int. J. Oncol.* 2015; 47(2):773-781.

[10] Orlando A, Linsalata M, Russo F. Antiproliferative effects on colon adenocarcinoma cells induced by co-administration of vitamin K1 and Lactobacillus rhamnosus GG. *Int. J. Oncol.* 2016; 48(6):2629-2638.

[11] Palermo A, Tuccinardi D, D'Onofrio L, Watanabe M, Maggi D, Maurizi AR, Greto V, Buzzetti R, Napoli N, Pozzilli P, Manfrini S. Vitamin K and osteoporosis: Myth or reality? *Metabolism.* 2017; 70: 57-71.

[12] Pearson DA. Bone health and osteoporosis: the role of vitamin K and potential antagonism by anticoagulants. *Nutr. Clin. Pract.* 2007; 22(5):517-544.

[13] Hamidi MS, Gajic-Veljanoski O, Cheung AM. Vitamin K and bone health. *J. Clin. Densitom.* 2013; 16(4):409-413.

[14] Azuma K, Inoue S. Multiple Modes of Vitamin K Actions in Aging-Related Musculoskeletal Disorders. *Int. J. Mol. Sci.* 2019; 20(11): 2844.

[15] Price PA, Urist MR, Otawar Y. Matrix Gla protein, a new gamma-carboxyglutamic acid-containing protein which is associated with the

organic matrix of bone. *Biochem. Biophys. Res. Commun.* 1983;117: 765–771.

[16] Wallin R, Schurgers LJ, Loeser RF. Biosynthesis of the vitamin K-dependent matrix Gla protein (MGP) in chondrocytes: A fetuin-MGP protein complex is assembled in vesicles shed from normal but not from osteoarthritic chondrocytes. *Osteoarthr. Cartil.* 2010; 18: 1096–1103.

[17] Rios H, Koushik SV, Wang H, Wang J, Zhou HM, Lindsley A, Rogers R, Chen Z, Maed M, Kruzynska-Frejtag A. Periostin null mice exhibit dwarfism, incisor enamel defects, and an early-onset periodontal disease-like phenotype. *Mol. Cell Biol.* 2005; 25: 11131–11144.

[18] Nakamura YS, Hakeda Y, Takakura N, Kameda T, Hamaguchi I.; Miyamoto T, Kakudo S, Nakano, T, Kumegawa M, Suda T. Tyro 3 receptor tyrosine kinase and its ligand, Gas6, stimulate the function of osteoclasts. *Stem Cells* 1998; 16: 229–238.

[19] Yu H, Wergedal JE, Zhao Y, Mohan S. Targeted disruption of TGFBI in mice reveals its role in regulating bone mass and bone size through periosteal bone formation. *Calcif. Tissue Int.* 2012; 91: 81–87.

[20] Tagariello A, Luther J, Streiter M, Didt-Koziel L, Wuelling M, Surmann-Schmitt C, Stock M, Adam N, Vortkamp A, Winterpacht A. Ucma–A novel secreted factor represents a highly specific marker for distal chondrocytes. *Matrix Biol.* 2008; 27: 3–11.

[21] Viegas CS, Simes DC, Laizé V, Williamson MK, Price PA, Cancela ML, Gla-rich protein (GRP), a new vitamin K-dependent protein identified from sturgeon cartilage and highly conserved in vertebrates. *J. Biol. Chem.* 2008; 283: 36655–36664.

[22] Rafael MS, Cavaco S, Viegas CS, Santos S, Ramos A, Willems, BA, Herfs M, Theuwissen E, Vermeer C, Simes DC. Insights into the association of Gla-rich protein and osteoarthritis, novel splice variants and γ-carboxylation status. *Mol. Nutr. Food Res.* 2014; 58: 1636–1646.

[23] Berkner KL, Pudota BN. Vitamin K-dependent carboxylation of the carboxylase. *Proc. Natl. Acad. Sci. USA* 1998; 95: 466–471.

[24] Weinreb M, Shinar D, Rodan GA. Different pattern of alkaline phosphatase, osteopontin, and osteocalcin expression in developing rat bone visualized by in situ hybridization. *J. Bone Miner. Res.* 1990; 5: 831–842.

[25] Szulc P, Chapu MC, Meunier PJ, Delmas PD. Serum undercarboxylated osteocalcin is a marker of the risk of hip fracture in elderly women. *J. Clin. Investig.* 1993; 91: 1769–1774.

[26] Azuma, K, Shiba S, Hasegawa T, Ikeda K, Urano T, Horie-Inoue, K, Ouchi Y, Amizuka N, Inoue S. Osteoblast-Specific γ-Glutamyl Carboxylase-Deficient Mice Display Enhanced Bone Formation With Aberrant Mineralization. *J. Bone Miner. Res.* 2015; 30: 1245–1254.

[27] Tanaka S, Miyazaki T, Uemura Y, Miyakawa N, Gorai I, Nakamura T, Fukunaga M, Ohashi Y, Ohta H, Mori S, Hagino H, Hosoi T, Sugimoto T, Itoi E, Orimo H, Shiraki M. Comparison of concurrent treatment with vitamin K 2 and risedronate compared with treatment with risedronate alone in patients with osteoporosis: Japanese Osteoporosis Intervention Trial-03. *J. Bone Miner. Metab.* 2017; 35(4): 385-395.

[28] Blumberg B, Sabbagh W Jr, Juguilon H, Bolado J Jr, van Meter CM, Ong ES, Evans RM. SXR, a novel steroid and xenobiotic-sensing nuclear receptor. *Genes Dev.* 1998; 12(20): 3195-205.

[29] Synold TW, Dussault I, Forman BM. The orphan nuclear receptor SXR coordinately regulates drug metabolism and efflux. *Nat. Med.* 2001;7(5): 584-590.

[30] Tabb MM, Sun A, Zhou C, Grün F, Errandi J, Romero K, Pham H, Inoue S, Mallick S, Lin M, Forman BM, Blumberg B. Vitamin K2 regulation of bone homeostasis is mediated by the steroid and xenobiotic receptor SXR. *J. Biol. Chem.* 2003; 278(45): 43919-43927.

[31] Suhara Y, Hanada N, Okitsu T, Sakai M, Watanabe M, Nakagawa K, Wada A, Takeda K, Takahashi K, Tokiwa H, Okano T. Structure-activity relationship of novel menaquinone-4 analogues: modification of the side chain affects their biological activities. *J. Med. Chem.* 2012; 55(4): 1553-1558.

[32] Otsuka M, Kato N, Ichimura T, Abe S, Tanaka Y, Taniguchi H, Hoshida Y, Moriyama M, Wang Y, Shao RX, Narayan D, Muroyama R, Kanai F, Kawabe T, Isobe T, Omata M. Vitamin K2 binds 17beta-hydroxysteroid dehydrogenase 4 and modulates estrogen metabolism. *Life Sci.* 2005; 76(21): 2473-2482.

[33] Karasawa S, Azuma M, Kasama T, Sakamoto S, Kabe Y, Imai T, Yamaguchi Y, Miyazawa K, Handa H. Vitamin K2 covalently binds to Bak and induces Bak-mediated apoptosis. *Mol. Pharmacol.* 2013; 83(3):613-620.

[34] Jilka RL, O'Brien CA, Roberson PK, Bonewald LF, Weinstein RS, Manolagas SC. Dysapoptosis of osteoblasts and osteocytes increases cancellous bone formation but exaggerates cortical porosity with age. *J. Bone Miner. Res.*; 29(1): 103-117.

[35] Vermeer C. Vitamin K: the effect on health beyond coagulation - an overview. *Food Nutr. Res.* 2012; 56.

[36] Evenepoel P, Claes K, Meijers B, Laurent M, Bammens B, Naesens M, Sprangers B, Pottel H, Cavalier E, Kuypers D. Poor Vitamin K Status Is Associated With Low Bone Mineral Density and Increased Fracture Risk in End-Stage Renal Disease. *J. Bone Miner. Res.* 2019; 34(2): 262-269.

[37] Fang Y, Hu C, Tao X, Wan Y, Tao F. Effect of vitamin K on bone mineral density: a meta-analysis of randomized controlled trials. *J. Bone Miner. MeTable* 2012; 30(1):60-68.

[38] Huang ZB, Wan SL, Lu YJ, Ning L, Liu C, Fan SW. Does vitamin K2 play a role in the prevention and treatment of osteoporosis for postmenopausal women: a meta-analysis of randomized controlled trials. *Osteoporos. Int.* 2015; 26(3): 1175-1186.

[39] Mott A, Bradley T, Wright K, Cockayne ES, Shearer MJ, Adamson J, Lanham-New SA, Torgerson DJ. Effect of vitamin K on bone mineral density and fractures in adults: an updated systematic review and meta-analysis of randomised controlled trials. *Osteoporos. Int.* 2019; 30(8): 1543-1559.

[40] Moore AE, Kim E, Dulnoan D, Dolan AL, Voong K, Ahmad I, Gorska R, Harrington DJ, Hampson G. Serum vitamin K 1 (phylloquinone) is

associated with fracture risk and hip strength in post-menopausal osteoporosis: A cross-sectional study. *Bone* 2020 Sep 10:115630.

[41] Weng SJ, Xie ZJ, Wu ZY, Yan DY, Tang JH, Shen ZJ, Li H, Bai BL, Boodhun V, Eric Dong XD, Yang L. Effects of combined menaquinone-4 and PTH 1-34 treatment on osetogenesis and angiogenesis in calvarial defect in osteopenic rats. *Endocrine.* 2019; 63(2): 376-384.

[42] Weng SJ, Yan DY, Gu LJ, Chen L, Xie ZJ, Wu ZY, Tang JH, Shen ZJ, Li H, Bai BL, Boodhun V, Yang L. Combined treatment with vitamin K2 and PTH enhanced bone formation in ovariectomized rats and increased differentiation of osteoblast in vitro. *Chem. Biol. Interact.* 2019; 300:101-110.

[43] Zhao B, Zhao W, Wang Y, Zhao Z, Zhao C, Wang S, Gao C. Prior administration of vitamin K2 improves the therapeutic effects of zoledronic acid in ovariectomized rats by antagonizing zoledronic acid-induced inhibition of osteoblasts proliferation and mineralization. *PLoS One* 2018; 13(8): e0202269.

[44] Muszyńska M, Ambrożewicz E, Gęgotek A, Grynkiewicz G, Skrzydlewska E. Protective Effects of Vitamin K Compounds on the Proteomic Profile of Osteoblasts under Oxidative Stress Conditions. *Molecules* 2020; 25(8):1990.

[45] Knapen MH, Drummen NE, Smit E, Vermeer C, Theuwissen E. Three-year low-dose menaquinone-7 supplementation helps decrease bone loss in healthy postmenopausal women. *Osteoporos. Int.* 2013; 24(9): 2499-2507.

[46] Cockayne S, Adamson J, Lanham-New S, Shearer MJ, Gilbody S, Torgerson DJ. Vitamin K and the prevention of fractures: systematic review and meta-analysis of randomized controlled trials. *Arch. Intern. Med.* 2006; 166(12):1256-1261.

[47] Fiordellisi W, White K, Schweizer M. A Systematic Review and Meta-analysis of the Association Between Vitamin K Antagonist Use and Fracture. *J. Gen. Intern. Med.* 2019; 34(2): 304-311.

[48] Sugiyama T. An update on hip fracture risk associated with anticoagulant therapy: warfarin versus direct oral anticoagulants. *Expert Opin. Drug Saf.* 2020:1-2.

[49] Oka H, Akune T, Muraki S, En-yo Y, Yoshida M, Saika A, Sasaki S, Nakamura K, Kawaguchi H, Yoshimura N. Association of low dietary vitamin K intake with radiographic knee osteoarthritis in the Japanese elderly population: dietary survey in a population-based cohort of the ROAD study. *Orthop. Sci.* 2009; 14(6):687-689.

[50] Misra D, Booth SL, Tolstykh I, Felson DT, Nevitt MC, Lewis CE, Torner J, Neogi T. Vitamin K deficiency is associated with incident knee osteoarthritis. *Am. J. Med.* 2013; 126(3): 243-248.

[51] Neogi T, Booth SL, Zhang YQ, Jacques PF, Terkeltaub R, Aliabadi P, Felson DT. Low vitamin K status is associated with osteoarthritis in the hand and knee. *Arthritis Rheum.* 2006; 54(4):1255-1261.

[52] Shea MK, Kritchevsky SB, Hsu FC, Nevitt M, Booth SL, Kwoh CK, McAlindon TE, Vermeer C, Drummen N, Harris TB, Womack C, Loeser RF; Health ABC Study. The association between vitamin K status and knee osteoarthritis features in older adults: the Health, Aging and Body Composition Study. *Osteoarthritis Cartilage* 2015; 23(3): 370-378.

[53] Neogi T, Felson DT, Sarno R, Booth SL. Vitamin K in hand osteoarthritis: results from a randomised clinical trial. *Ann. Rheum. Dis.* 2008; 67(11):1570-1573.

[54] Rafael MS, Cavaco S, Viegas CS, Santos S, Ramos A, Willems BA, Herfs M, Theuwissen E, Vermeer C, Simes DC. Insights into the association of Gla-rich protein and osteoarthritis, novel splice variants and γ-carboxylation status. *Mol. Nutr. Food Res.* 2014; 58(8):1636-1646.

[55] van Ballegooijen AJ, van Putten SR, Visser M, Beulens JW, Hoogendijk EO. Vitamin K status and physical decline in older adults-The Longitudinal Aging Study Amsterdam. *Maturitas.* 2018;113:73-79.

INDEX

A

acid, 84, 107, 111, 115, 119
activity level, 105
adverse effects, 38, 48, 59, 64, 87
age, 9, 10, 11, 12, 13, 14, 15, 16, 17, 18, 19, 20, 21, 22, 23, 24, 25, 26, 27, 28, 29, 30, 31, 32, 33, 85, 100, 105, 111, 118
age-related diseases, 85, 100
alkaline phosphatase, 94, 117
antitumor, ix, 82, 86, 90, 95, 97
apoptosis, ix, 82, 86, 87, 88, 91, 93, 94, 95, 96, 98, 99, 100, 101, 108, 111, 115, 118
assessment, viii, 2, 7, 9, 33, 36, 37, 38, 39, 40, 41, 42, 43, 44, 45, 46, 47

B

bacteria, 84, 101, 106
bias, viii, 2, 7, 9, 34, 35, 36, 37, 38, 39, 40, 41, 42, 43, 44, 45, 46, 47, 60, 61
bioavailability, 99
biomarkers, 23, 56, 108
biosynthesis, 115
blood, viii, ix, 2, 22, 23, 24, 26, 27, 31, 33, 38, 57, 61, 64, 65, 83, 89, 90, 104, 105
bone, vii, ix, 4, 28, 56, 82, 85, 87, 90, 92, 94, 95, 97, 98, 99, 100, 101, 104, 105, 107, 108, 109, 110, 111, 112, 114, 115, 116, 117, 118, 119
bone cancer, 92
bone form, ix, x, 82, 104, 110, 116, 118, 119
bone marrow, 104, 107, 111, 112
bone mass, 105, 109, 116
bone metabolism, vii, ix, 90, 94, 95, 104, 109, 114
bone mineral content, 56
bone mineral densisty, 104
bone resorption, 105, 108
bone tumors, ix, 82, 95
bones, ix, 82, 105, 107

C

calcification, 85, 100, 106, 107, 113

calcium, ix, 4, 6, 21, 22, 23, 25, 28, 29, 31, 33, 54, 64, 82, 84, 90, 94, 98, 105, 107, 109, 111
cancer, ix, 82, 86, 88, 90, 91, 100
cardiovascular disease, 85, 105, 106
cardiovascular diseases, 85
cardiovascular system, 98
cartilage, 85, 107, 112, 113, 114, 116
cell cycle, 86, 88, 89, 92, 95
cell death, ix, 82, 87, 88, 98, 101
cell differentiation, 87, 93, 99
cell invasion, 93
cell line, ix, 82, 88, 91, 92, 93, 94, 97, 98, 100, 102, 115
cell lines, ix, 82, 91, 93, 94, 100, 102, 115
chemiluminescence, 13, 15, 16, 19
cholecalciferol, 6, 21, 23, 28, 29, 43, 78, 89
clinical trials, viii, 2, 7, 8, 21, 35, 65, 94, 114
compounds, 83, 86, 89, 95, 105, 111
computer, 36, 37, 38, 40, 41, 42, 43, 45
consumption, 10, 11, 14, 16, 61, 87
control group, viii, 2, 27, 54, 55, 58, 60, 64, 111, 113
controlled studies, vii, 2, 5, 61, 63
controlled trials, 5, 47, 118, 119

D

defects, x, 104, 110, 112, 116
deficiency, vii, 2, 3, 4, 5, 6, 7, 8, 10, 11, 15, 16, 17, 20, 21, 22, 24, 25, 30, 31, 33, 48, 52, 61, 62, 64, 65, 66, 67, 68, 70, 74, 76, 85, 99, 105, 106, 108, 115, 120
detection, 36, 37, 38, 39, 40, 41, 42, 43, 44, 45, 46, 47
diabetes, 55, 64, 65, 85, 90
dietary supplements, 6, 29, 82
diseases, x, 85, 104, 105, 114

E

economic status, 10, 17, 62
evidence, vii, 2, 4, 60, 61, 64, 82, 85, 95, 96, 98, 100, 110
exposure, 9, 10, 11, 12, 18, 61, 86, 87, 89, 93, 105

F

food, 3, 62, 63, 84, 101, 106
formation, 88, 105, 108, 110
fractures, x, 84, 97, 104, 105, 109, 110, 112, 114, 118, 119

G

gene expression, 64, 87, 89
genes, ix, 82, 91, 92, 97, 104, 108
gestation, 16, 17, 18, 21, 22, 23, 24, 25, 26, 27, 28, 29, 30, 31, 32, 33, 65
gestational age, 48
gestational diabetes, viii, 2, 4, 6, 10, 55, 56, 61, 64
growth, ix, 56, 82, 86, 87, 88, 93, 95, 102, 104, 107, 115

H

health, 4, 37, 39, 64, 85, 94, 97, 98, 99, 100, 101, 105, 114, 115, 118
heterogeneity, viii, 2, 8, 48, 49, 52, 55, 58, 65
homeostasis, ix, 90, 100, 104, 108, 117
human, 84, 85, 87, 88, 89, 91, 92, 96, 97, 98, 99, 100, 101, 106, 108, 111, 115
human body, 84, 106
human health, 99, 100
hydroxycholecalciferols, 6
hypercalcemia, 54, 60, 90

hypertension, 4, 10, 13, 22, 48

I

in vitro, ix, 83, 97, 104, 108, 110, 119
in vivo, ix, 93, 94, 97, 104, 108, 110
India, 1, 10, 11, 12, 13, 14, 23, 26, 61, 70, 76
inflammation, x, 92, 97, 104, 109
inflammatory bowel disease, 97
inflammatory mediators, 56
inhibition, 88, 91, 92, 93, 111, 113, 119
intervention, 36, 37, 38, 39, 40, 41, 43, 45, 46, 63, 64, 83

L

lesions, 112
level of education, 12
ligand, 108, 116
lipoproteins, 106
liquid chromatography, 16, 19
liver, 3, 84, 86, 89, 90, 106
longitudinal study, 16
lymphatic system, 106

M

management, v, vii, viii, 1, 2, 3, 7, 8, 21, 96
measurement, 7, 21, 22, 23, 24, 25, 26, 27, 28, 29, 30, 31, 32, 33, 36, 40, 41, 66
measurements, 27, 37, 38, 41
mellitus, 4, 10, 55, 56, 64, 90
menadione, 83, 84, 87, 88, 98, 101, 105, 106
metabolism, vii, ix, 3, 63, 82, 85, 90, 94, 95, 104, 105, 107, 108, 109, 115, 118
migration, ix, 82, 88, 92, 95
mineralization, ix, 85, 94, 104, 107, 111, 119

musculoskeletal, x, 95, 104, 105, 108, 114

N

necrosis, ix, 82, 88, 98, 101
negative relation, 112
neonates, viii, 2, 4, 27, 57, 64, 65

O

osteoarthritis, x, 85, 90, 96, 104, 116, 120
osteoblasts, ix, 88, 101, 104, 107, 108, 111, 118, 119
osteoporosis, x, 85, 90, 98, 104, 105, 106, 109, 110, 111, 114, 115, 117, 118, 119
osteosarcoma progression, 82, 93, 97
oxidative stress, 87, 91, 92, 97, 101

P

parathyroid hormone, 13, 54
participants, 5, 6, 8, 11, 14, 21, 22, 23, 24, 25, 26, 27, 28, 29, 30, 31, 36, 37, 38, 39, 40, 41, 42, 43, 44, 45, 46, 47, 49, 52, 53, 55, 57, 58, 60
perinatal care, 6
pigmentation, 3, 9, 20, 62, 65
placebo, 5, 21, 23, 24, 25, 26, 27, 28, 29, 32, 33, 36, 41, 48, 55, 60, 63, 65, 111
population, viii, 2, 4, 48, 61, 63, 106, 109, 110, 120
pregnancy, vii, 2, 4, 5, 6, 7, 8, 9, 10, 13, 21, 33, 36, 41, 42, 48, 52, 62, 63, 64, 65, 66, 67, 68, 69, 70, 71, 72, 73, 74, 75, 76, 77, 78, 79
pregnancy/drug therapy, 6
pregnant women, v, vii, 1, 3, 4, 5, 6, 8, 44, 48, 49, 54, 61, 63, 65, 66, 67, 69, 70, 71, 72, 73, 74, 76
preparation, iv

prevalence, v, vii, 1, 3, 4, 5, 6, 7, 8, 9, 10, 11, 12, 13, 14, 15, 16, 17, 18, 19, 20, 48, 52, 61, 62, 65, 68, 69, 70, 71, 72
prevention, vii, x, 6, 64, 65, 97, 98, 104, 110, 111, 118, 119
proliferation, 89, 91, 92, 93, 95, 96, 98, 107, 119
prostate cancer, 96, 97
prostate carcinoma, 98
protective role, 85, 88
proteins, ix, 82, 84, 85, 94, 104, 105, 107, 113

R

random numbers, 36, 38
receptor, ix, 64, 89, 90, 91, 92, 98, 100, 104, 108, 116, 117
risk, viii, x, 2, 4, 7, 9, 20, 36, 37, 38, 39, 40, 41, 42, 43, 44, 45, 46, 47, 55, 56, 60, 61, 62, 64, 65, 85, 98, 104, 105, 106, 108, 109, 110, 112, 114, 117, 119, 120

S

serum, vii, x, 2, 6, 15, 17, 54, 59, 60, 104, 109, 110, 111, 114
side chain, 83, 84, 105, 106, 117
signal transduction, 85
signaling pathway, 91, 98, 99
skin, 3, 9, 14, 15, 61, 65, 89
standard deviation, 8, 49, 58
supplementation, vii, 2, 4, 5, 6, 8, 9, 16, 35, 39, 48, 49, 55, 56, 58, 59, 61, 62, 63, 65, 67, 77, 85, 99, 109, 112, 113, 119
synergistic effect, x, 94, 104, 111
synthesis, 3, 64, 65, 84, 94, 99
synthetic analogues, 84

T

therapeutic effect, 111, 119
therapeutic use, 6
transcription, ix, 104, 108
treatment, vii, viii, x, 2, 5, 39, 41, 42, 44, 47, 49, 50, 54, 55, 57, 60, 63, 64, 82, 84, 88, 91, 92, 93, 95, 98, 104, 108, 110, 113, 117, 118, 119
trial, viii, 2, 6, 8, 21, 22, 23, 24, 25, 27, 28, 29, 30, 31, 32, 38, 39, 40, 41, 42, 43, 56, 65, 77, 113, 120
tumor, 93, 98, 100
tumor growth, 93

U

underlying mechanisms, vii, ix, 82, 96, 111

V

vitamin D, v, vii, ix, 1, 3, 4, 5, 6, 7, 8, 9, 10, 11, 12, 13, 14, 15, 16, 17, 18, 19, 20, 21, 22, 23, 24, 25, 26, 27, 28, 29, 30, 31, 32, 33, 35, 39, 48, 49, 52, 53, 54, 55, 56, 57, 58, 59, 60, 61, 63, 64, 65, 66, 67, 68, 69, 70, 71, 72, 73, 74, 75, 76, 77, 78, 79, 82, 89, 90, 91, 92, 93, 94, 95, 97, 98, 101, 102, 113
vitamin D deficiency, v, vii, 1, 4, 5, 6, 7, 8, 9, 10, 11, 16, 20, 21, 48, 52, 61, 64, 65, 67, 68, 69, 70, 71, 72, 73, 74, 75, 77, 78
vitamin K, v, vii, ix, 82, 83, 84, 85, 86, 87, 89, 94, 95, 96, 97, 98, 99, 100, 101, 102, 103, 104, 105, 106, 107, 108, 109, 110, 111, 112, 113, 114, 115, 116, 117, 118, 119, 120
vitamins, vii, ix, 82, 94, 95, 97, 99, 100, 105, 106, 109